W.

Making you Healthy, Happy and Thin is what happens here

Thin You, Thin Me and the Power of Chi

by

Allison Kummery & Martin Katz, MD

Hannah Davis & Amanda Main
Wes Bagby & Shane
Charles (Chaz) William Glunk II

Cover photo by TomShanePhotos.com

Printed in the United States of America

This book contains the opinions and ideas of its writers. It is sold with the understanding that the writers and publisher may or may not be engaged in rendering medical, health, or any other kind of professional health care advice. The reader should consult with a health care professional before adopting the recommendations and conclusions in this book. The writers and publisher disclaim all responsibility for any liability, loss, or risk, personal or otherwise, which is incurred as a consequence, directly or indirectly, of the use and application of any of the content contained in this book.

ISBN: 978-0-9844664-3-6

Library of Congress Control Number: 2011903895

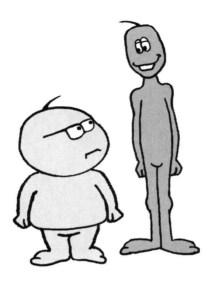

The distilled wisdom of many sources on healthful living make up this book. The combination of practical lore and pithy humor make it an easy read, but an essential one, nevertheless. Worth taking to heart — and brain, and stomach and other vital parts.

—Norman Julian, writer and publisher

INTRODUCTION

Once in awhile a special book offers sane solutions for serious health and personal problems; solutions that will heal you and make you happier. "Thin You, Thin Me and the Power of Chi" is healing because three foundations for good health came together; Asian tradition, western science, and the Spirit of Loving Kindness. Here are solutions for the 90% of us who don't breathe properly for optimal health; the 80% who require expensive and annoying dental treatments because of improper oral hygiene; the half of adult America that's overweight or obese and needs to get thin again. How to take better care of your heart and head/brain/mind so they take better care of you also is in the book. Lest we forget, there's a recipe for making your very own miracle.

This "Chi" book is easy to read, but read it slowly so you can peel some love off its pages; love being the best emotional bonding material available to craft together 24,241 healing words. Stories in the book were written by people who have struggled physically, spiritually, or mentally along the path to wellness. They know there is no miracle drug or predetermined formula that will make everyone feel better. They know that our well being comes from within. Healing a body starts with healing a heart, a mind, and a soul. There is no one approach to wellness that applies to all of us, but many pathways to better health do exist, and many of them happen to be in this book. You can apply one or more to your life today to feel better, maybe not tomorrow, but surely the day after tomorrow.

We believe that special books pretty much write themselves, but the surprise of surprises to us was that the soul of the book, the real power of Chi, was a gift to both readers and writers that came from the Spirit of Loving Kindness. Her healing touch will rock your reality, and make you smile.

CONTENTS

I. Healing

II. Exercise

III. Weight

IV. Food

V. Dental perfection

VI. Miracles & more

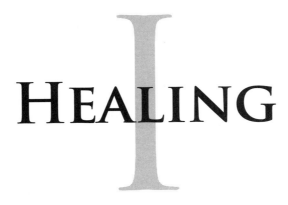

HEALING

How to harness the power of chi

Have you ever felt energy in a room? In the moments before ringing in the new year, while watching a sunrise, or the birthing of a baby? What is life? What is it that is born in the womb and leaves our bodies when we exhale for the last time? This is the powerful, vibrant, encompassing energy called Chi. It is a philosophy that can guide us toward better health and happiness.

Chi can be compared to an electrical charge that connects everything in life. It is like an invisible web of force. When the web is touched, it sends out a vibration that affects everything, like the ripples that follow after a stone is thrown into a pond. When our Chi is in balance, our pond is placid and calm. When something happens in our lives that throws us off balance, our waters begin to churn. The result can be good or bad, but if we understand this we may prevent or ease an undesirable outcome. The concept of Chi can be stated simply. There is balance in everything, including us. When we become imbalanced, we are more susceptible to health problems.

When we are in balance, we feel more at peace with ourselves and our surroundings.

Breathe the breath of life

We can achieve inner harmony by cultivating Chi through meditation, physical movement, and breathing techniques. Studies have shown that 90 percent of Americans breathe from the upper respiratory system only. The upper respiratory system activates the "fight or flight" part of our nervous system. When we breathe in our upper lungs alone, our stress levels increase.

If I had to limit my advice on healthier living to just one tip,
it would be simply to learn how to breathe correctly.
—Andrew Weil, MD

Chi breathing utilizes the entire respiratory system, and activates the "rest and digest" part of our nervous system. Correct breathing increases our energy levels and healing capabilities. It assists with removing toxins from the body and negative thinking from the mind. Blood circulation increases, blood pressure improves, the immune system gets a boost. Oxygen into our blood stream increases. Mental awareness grows. Even the enjoyment of sex is heightened. Just ten minutes of Chi breathing every day can have a positive effect on overall health and happiness.

Chi breathing can be practiced anywhere. For optimal results, choose a quiet place with fresh air. Sit upright, either on a chair with feet planted, or on the floor using a cushion with legs crossed. Being comfortable is important. Your spine should be upright, without being rigid.

Begin by breathing normally. Notice where your breath is traveling in your body. Your mindfulness will cause your breath to slow and your mind to quiet. After a few minutes, you will be ready to begin the methods listed below. They should be performed in a calm, relaxed way. Adjust the length of these practices to whatever feels comfortable to you.

Breathing in, I calm body and mind,
Breathing out, I Smile.
Dwelling in the present moment,
I know this is the only moment.

—Thich Nhat Hanh

LOTUS FLOWER BREATHING: The first Chi breathing method is a good way to learn lower lung breathing. It is practiced lying down, with knees bent and feet planted on the floor. STEP 1: Lay on your back and place your hands on your stomach. Close your eyes. Breathe in and out of your nose for a couple of minutes. Allow your belly to rise and fall with your breath. Breaths should be easy but full.

STEP 2: Inhale through your nose, allowing your belly to rise. Exhale through your mouth. Continue for two minutes. Relax your body while you breathe. STEP 3: Inhale through your nose and hold your breath for three seconds. Exhale through your mouth, allowing all the air to move gently out of your body. After exhaling, close your mouth and hold for three seconds. Repeat for three minutes. If holding your breath makes you feel tense, try shortening the length of the holds. If you still feel tense, go back to practicing step 2.

FLYING DRAGON CHI: STEP 1: Sit in a chair or on the floor with your back straight. Inhale through your nose and exhale through your mouth for two minutes. STEP 2: Inhale deeper and feel your stomach rise with your breath. Exhale slowly and completely. Continue this breathing pattern for two minutes.

STEP 3: While inhaling deeply, raise your arms from your sides to above your head and lace your fingers together. Hold your breath for three seconds. Exhale completely and lower your hands gently onto your lap. Pause, and hold your out-breath for three seconds. Repeat for four minutes. When you get familiar with this method, skip step 1.

GOLDEN CRANE CHI: STEP 1: Sit upright on the floor or in a chair. Inhale through your nose and exhale through your mouth. Repeat for two minutes. STEP 2: Raise your arms out to your sides like wings. Turn your wrists up. Inhaling, raise your arms as you count four seconds. Turn your wrists downward. Exhaling, gently lower your arms back down as you count four seconds. Repeat this 4:6:4 pattern for four minutes.

> *For breath is life, and if you breathe well*
> *you will live long on earth.*
> —Sanskrit Proverb

Figure 8 chi

This is one of the simpler methods, but effective with the added feature of closing your eyes. While sitting with your back straight, close your eyes and breathe in through your nose for eight seconds – again breathing deeply to fill up your belly.

Keeping your eyes closed, exhale through your mouth for eight seconds. Repeat for five minutes always in a relaxed, calm way.

Dragon fire chi

One of the more advance methods but it is also one of the most effective methods you can try. While standing up, clench and tighten all of the muscles in your body except stomach and inhale deeply through the nose inflating your stomach with air.

After inhaling, relax muscles while tightening only your abdominal muscles and exhale deeply and powerfully as if you were trying to blow someone over. Repeat for 5 minutes.

You may want to start out by simply exhaling deeply and slowly build up how forcefully you want to exhale until you are comfortable. Do not hyper-ventilate yourself. Do it in a calm, relaxed way.

Crouching tiger chi

Another advanced method that brings wonderful results. On the ground on all fours, deeply, slowly inhale through the nose. As you exhale through the mouth, lean your body forward until your chin is just inches above the ground.

Hold for three seconds. Then inhale deeply and slowly while gently returning to your original position. Repeat for five minutes. During inhalation, visualize that you are filling up your stomach (your inflatable tire) with air. Exhale through your mouth. You may want to start out with normal inhaling and exhaling for the first two minutes to get used to the flow of the movement.

Doctor's Advisory

by Andrew Weil, MD, On-line newsletter, 6/9/2003

"Today I want you to notice how you're breathing throughout the day. This simple activity can tell you the state of your nervous system – and by learning to control your breathing, you can influence the regulation of your heart rate, blood pressure, circulation, and digestion.

"Since your have more control over exhalation, focusing on this part of your breathing is one good way of learning how to breathe deeper. Use the muscles between your ribs to squeeze air out of your lungs – when you move more air out, you will automatically take more air in. As you breathe in and out, think of the cycle as having no beginning or end. Practice this exercise as often as you like, but I recommend doing it at least once each day."

Tai chi

The gentle forms of Tai chi use dance-like flowing movements that require concentration, resulting in reduced stress and more calm. Movements are graceful, one flowing into the next without pause. There is a constant state of relaxed motion. Call it slow dancing or meditation in motion, Tai chi is beautiful to watch and is helpful in treating serious illness.

In April 2011, researchers at Harvard reported that Tai chi improves the quality of life in people with heart failure. Historically, patients with heart failure were advised not to exercise. During the 1980s, medical opinion viewed physical exercise as something to avoid because patients with heart failure were considered too frail.

The Harvard study found that heart patients practicing Tai chi had greater improvements in quality of life than non-participating heart patients. This included increased confidence to perform exercises and greater feelings of well-being. The researchers noted that Tai chi may be beneficial for hypertension, balance problems, and impaired exercise capacity.

Tai chi decreases anxiety, enhances vigor, and improves mood. It's certainly a safe alternative to more intense exercising like jogging. Many types of Tai chi workouts are gentle and safe for seniors who may otherwise not exercise. The body/mind flow of energy in rhythmic patterns of movement is sometimes set to music. These motions are coordinated with Chi breathing to help achieve a sense of inner calm. Concentrating on the movements allows us to live in the present moment. Focusing on the present moment leads to positive thinking with no space left in our minds for negative thoughts.

Tai chi also is recommended by health care professionals as a safe program for long term fitness and self discipline. It is also employed as an adjunct treatment for arthritis, low bone density, Parkinson's disease, sleep problems, stroke and breast cancer.

CHAKRAS 7 points of life

Do you believe in angels? Does prayer have a place in your life? What about your soul? When was the last time you peeked into something beyond the visible and the obvious, like your soul, or for that matter, your chakras?

Seven invisible health promoting forces may be in all of us, but only a few know much about them. Yet these seven Chakras could be as important as our other spiritual or metaphysical connections. Read now about chakras and how they may influence the quality of your life.

Chakras are believed to be vortexes of energy contained within and about our bodies and important to general health and well being. Each is located at specific points that generally correspond with the spine and has a specific role in influencing or controlling important aspects of our lives.

When a chakra is strong, that aspect of life tends to go well. When it weakens, it can be compared to the dimming of a light bulb at a time when more illumination is necessary. These Seven Points of Life could be the architecture to our soul. Learning how to balance them may enhance your life.

The root chakra influences careers, money, our sense of belonging, and our relationship to the physical world. It is located at the base of the spine. When we are stuck in a stressful job or plagued by too much debt, the root chakra may be weak. This can lead to additional problems like overeating or not eating enough, thereby making us uncomfortable in our own skin. Being overly attached to the physical world (hoarding) is an example of an imbalanced root chakra. When this chakra is strong, we enjoy our work, feel a sense of connection to others, and have a healthy relationship with money.

The sacral (sex) chakra is associated with feelings, desire, emotions, imagination. It helps determine how we interact with others, our sense of self worth, and our creativity. The sacral chakra allows us to be sensual, enthusiastic, curious and creative. This chakra is located about two inches below the navel.

An unawake sacral chakra makes it difficult to express true sensual nature. If blocked, the consequences can be an emotional imbalance, manipulative relationships, obsession with sex, fear of sex, or a paucity of energy or enthusiasm for it. A faltering sex chakra could result in impotence, frigidity, high blood pressure; perhaps even a seat on a government advisory panel.

A balanced sacral chakra is cultivated through activities that allow us to enjoy our bodies such as dance, massage, music, good food. When two people make love, the lights from their sex chakras merge and a beautiful aura surrounds them, especially so if they are "in" love. A forest full of roses and trees bearing delicious fruits is where we dwell when this chakra is healthy and we embrace love in our lives.

The heart chakra is the emotional center for warmth, radiance, and the feeling of pure love. Of all the chakras, it's the most precious because pure love, absent of egoism, calculation, demands, is the most important quality a human being can possess. This chakra is essential to spiritual development. It helps us feel the warmth (or chill) emanating from other people. It sends and receives love. An unbalanced or weakened heart chakra inhibits love. We may see the other person as a possession, or someone to dominate.

The crown chakra at the top of the head is our connection to the divine. When you feel connected to a higher power, or even the better nature of yourself, the crown chakra is strong. You know what you need to know, and understand what needs to be understood. A strong crown chakra allows you to see the big picture. Not much about life is mysterious. The universal plan is clear. There's an appreciation of others, and a powerful attachment to love. An inability to connect to the spiritual side of life may indicate a problem with the crown chakra.

The throat chakra when healthy enables clear communications. It relates to our ability to be heard and also listen. It helps us express feelings, and maintain relationships. When we feel no one cares about our opinion, and we withdraw, our throat chakra may be blocked. We may talk too much, or catch a sore throat.

The power chakra, located in the solar plexus, helps us gain confidence and health. When this chakra is strong, our self-esteem is high. We speak our mind and encourage others to do so. We strive to help make the world a better place. When we struggle with self-esteem issues and feelings of unworthiness, when we are indecisive or feel victimized by random circumstance, this chakra may have weakened.

The Third Eye (brow) chakra is a somewhat mystical concept. Some believe it is the gateway to higher consciousness and enlightenment. It is related to imagination, insight, intuition and an ability to perceive clearly. It helps thoughts become actions. It draws energy into the brain. It helps us express our feelings, and maintain relationships.

This chakra is located between the eyebrows on the forehead. It can absorb energy from the environment and from other people.

When you pick up good or bad "vibes" from another person, you know this chakra is working well. If you want to know more about chakras, contact your neighborhood Yoga specialist.

Yoga for every body

Over 10 million Americans have practiced Yoga and received health benefits from this 5,000 year old gift from Asia. They learned how to move the body in ways that improve flexibility, balance and strength. Most classes include breathing and meditation techniques.

Yoga stretches muscles and the soft tissues, creating a sense of fluidity in the body. You can expect to become more flexible and enjoy other physical health benefits within eight weeks. Like Einstein's theory that matter is energy, Yoga proposes that we are made of more than just physical bodies. There are additional mental and spiritual aspects to us. One way to think of this is to imagine our bodies being layered like an onion, interconnected and influencing one another.

The energy body consists of currents of consciousness similar to the meridians in acupuncture. They may clog, dry up, or overflow as we move through life. Making positive lifestyle changes through Yoga allows us to untie the "knots" of our lives.

One way to visualize what the energy body looks like is to think of it as an internal sun. As we age, our energy sources reduce. Harnessing the energy of our internal sun may alleviate ailments such as chronic fatigue. Yoga also works powerfully at the psychological level and can help alleviate depression, anxiety and mental instability.

Strength and endurance come along with improved muscle tone. Some Yoga poses, Downward Dog, Upward Dog, build upper body strength. Standing poses build strength in hamstrings, quadriceps and abdominal muscles. Better posture comes with increased flexibility and strength.

Some beginners at Yoga report less stress in their lives and feel more relaxed after only a few sessions. Yoga styles often depend on deep breathing techniques that focus the mind on the breath, making us calm. This may relieve depression because it boosts oxygen levels in the brain.

Generally Yogis practice between 4 and 7 a.m. in quiet environments that are free of distraction. Little or no food is in their bellies. The heart benefits too. Yoga lowers blood pressure and slows the heart rate. With its popularity so high, the National Institute of Health has funded research on possible benefits from the practice of Yoga (learning and memory, slowing the aging process, increasing energy levels).

Potential Yoga benefits for Every Body include better health and more strength; a clear, calm, well-disciplined mind; an intellect sharp as a razor and as strong as steel; and a heart filled with love and compassion.

Acupuncture

Acupuncture is a good way to understand how Chi energy works. It utilizes body energy points for pain treatment and recovery. Acupuncture helps to balance the flow of Chi in body pathways called meridians. It involves the insertion of extremely thin needles into the skin at specific points along these meridians. When symptoms are determined, needles are applied to the energy points associated with areas of body weakness. Acupuncture stimulates nerves, muscles and connective tissue to increase the body's natural painkillers and circulation.

About 15 million Americans have undergone acupuncture treatments in the past 30 years. The World Health Organization has approved the procedure to treat dozens of ailments including back pain, migraines, depression, allergies, respiratory ailments, hypertension, alcoholism, substance abuse and weight management.

Acupuncture is considered an adjunct therapy, but not a wonder cure for weight issues. When accompanied by healthful lifestyle changes, it may assist with weight loss. Dieters are treated for both physiological and psychological aspects, and have reported improvements in digestion, emotional health and appetite reduction. One study reported that acupuncture patients lost three times more weight than its control group.

Acupressure uses the same pressure points and meridians as acupuncture, but instead of needles it utilizes fingertips to press healing points that activate the curative abilities of the body.

When acupressure points are stimulated, they release muscle tension, promote blood circulation and strengthen the flow of Chi. Acupressure can be a self treatment to relieve stress, tension and pain.

Meditation

Meditation may be the only intentional human act which in the bottom line is not about improving yourself, or trying to get somewhere else emotionally or physically, but simply to realize where you already are, and staying for awhile. That seems to be its value, and probably it's something we should all do periodically for its own sake, because a day's worth of stress can be wiped out with about 15 minutes of meditation.

Whether you are anxious, tense, worried, or stressed out, meditation can bring inner peace and calm. Meditation lowers stress levels and blood pressure. It increases energy levels, memory, learning and creativity. Our muscles relax. We sleep with peace of mind. If those are not enough reasons to try meditating, how about simply to bring more joy into your life?

One good idea to get started meditating is with a group or class because meditation may feel uncomfortable at first. Having a support network of like-minded people can help keep you on track whenever you wonder whether meditating is your cup of emotional tea. Even if you don't actually speak to anyone in the group, there is something special about a few people getting together to meditate. If the group chats, you can listen to the challenges of others and learn how they cope.

Otherwise, meditate anytime you want to calm down and de-clutter your mind. Do it at home where no equipment is needed and any amount of time will do. Prepare a meditating space where you place a favorite chair or cushion or whatever is comfortable, but not too comfortable. You don't want to fall asleep unless that is the goal of your meditation.

Once the right spot is chosen, meditate there every day to train your mind and body to relax as soon as you enter this space. Keep this special area free of clutter. Make it an easy place to feel at peace and serene in your body.

Many who routinely meditate awaken earlier than the rest of the household, before disruptions or distractions can occur. Start your meditation sitting, spine straight, vertebra stacked on vertebra, head floating, shoulders in line with hips, nose in line with navel. This posture allows you to be upright with the least amount of effort. If sitting, keep feet flat on the floor. If on a cushion or the floor, you can sit cross-legged or kneeling. Whatever you do, get as comfortable as possible so circulation continues to flow smoothly to all areas of the body.

Begin meditating with eyes closed by relaxing each body part individually, starting with the toes. Then move, body part by body part, all the way to the scalp, including the muscles of the face and your tongue.

With eyes closed, observe your breath; then focus on it. Feeling the natural flow of your breath in a relaxed state will allow your mind to settle. If your mind begins to drift away from breathing, gently nudge it back into focus. Mental focusing leaves little room for dwelling on stress producers like job, money, health, relationships.

When you wish to come out of the meditation, take notice again of your body parts. Perhaps wiggle your fingers and toes, open your eyes, and stretch. Then continue the day in a positive frame of mind.

Asthma, allergies, anxiety disorders, binge eating, depression, high blood pressure, pain, sleep problems, substance abuse can lessen with meditation. Medical experts consider meditating to be a safe, complementary addition to conventional medicine, and free. That alone makes it easy to feel good about. Various types of meditation follow.

Mindful meditation focuses on breathing. You listen to the sounds of your breath inhaling and exhaling, or simply count each exhale. When you reach 50, reverse the count. Mentally scan your body. Become aware of the feelings and sensations, perhaps the pain, in various body parts. Bring your breath into those places as a healing agent.

Mantra meditation is you repeating the same soothing word or phrase that may or may not have any particular meaning to you. You focus on a sound like "ahhhoom", allowing it to fill your mind. This can produce a state of relaxation all by itself.

Tai chi & Yoga use meditation techniques as part of their unique approach to health enhancement. Walking meditation combines the benefits of physical exercise with mental relaxation. The common thread to all meditations is the ability to quiet the mind enough to sense the peace that is within. It is a peace of mind too often ignored as we get caught up in complicated living issues; bill paying, legal and in-law issues, or tonight's quarrel.

These thoughts focus on the past and the future. Meditation keeps us in the here and now. The gifts that meditation brings usually don't happen during the meditation itself, but arrive throughout the day. They present themselves as grace during times of crisis and serenity in times of struggle. Perhaps for the first time we can touch that spark of divinity within us, and release all judgment of ourselves and others.

Without an occasional touch of peace and harmony in our lives, we can become mentally fatigued, with weakened chakras or a compromised immune system. We unconsciously allow sickness to take control when it is the enhancement of health we need to encourage via meditation, nutritious foods, exercise and enough quality sleep.

Our bodies respond to real or imagined stress in the same manner, without discrimination. Meditation helps us see that at least for right now, all is well. Right now we are at a place where our needs are met. We see things clearly. We look at life as a place of love, not fear. Meditation takes us to this place.

All the things I really like to do are either immoral, illegal, or fattening.
—Alexander Woollcott

Dieting is not a piece of cake.
—Unknown

If food is your best friend, it's also your worst enemy.
—Grandpa Jones (1978)

People say that losing weight is no walk in the park. When I hear that I think, yeah, that's the problem.
—Chris Adams

EXERCISE

Well'th: An investment in YOUR HEALTH

by Martin Katz, MD

While sitting with a good friend eating lunch (healthy, of course), I came up with the idea of well'th. To my surprise and disappointment it had already been used. But is this such a surprise? We know on some level that if we are healthier, we are likely to be wealthier. With the cost of medicines, doctor visits, diagnostic testing, hospital stays, surgeries, therapy etc. the more we can minimize, the more likely we are to stay out of monetary purgatory. The most common reason for bankruptcy in the United States is medical costs. And most of these folks had filed with insurance companies.

Sure, not all medical problems are preventable, but a lot are, especially diabetes. And this is not even taking into account the folks who did not go bankrupt but had to contend with stressors due to exorbitant costs of medicines and medical testing. So come on, give yourself a hug and start investing in yourself. Not only will you reap the long term benefits of living longer, you'll have a better time enjoying the ride.

Just imagine more energy, less anxiety/depression, less shortness of breath, and improved health. Think about it. You don't put leaded gasoline in your car anymore, why continue to put crap into your body?

From a medical standpoint, our bodies have essential highways and roads. If we lay down roads made from low quality products that were not designed to last, they won't. Then when navigating over that bridge or highway that we expect/assume will support us, low and behold it doesn't. We crash, die and burn in the process.

Yet we consume junky foods, trying to build and maintain a healthy body that we assume/expect will keep on ticking without regard to proper maintenance. When our bodies don't work as we think they should, we visit the doctor expecting miracles without putting in any thought to how we could prevent or improve the issue.

Unfortunately, most doctors are too busy to be able to sit down and go through a thorough evaluation of our lifestyle. Even worse, some doctors don't know how to ffectively do this, or don't have the support necessary to get patients going in the right direction.

Like the scenario above, we make a mistake when we are lucky enough to survive a huge pothole in the road, and take the car in to get fixed and serviced, without improving the road. Too often we treat our cars, houses, even our wardrobes, better than we treat ourselves.

It is definitely time to make a change and apply some of the good news out there. We can make a positive difference in our lives by taking the advice in this book and investing in better health.

I've been privileged to be the physician of some incredible patients. Many difficult cases, some sad, others with happier endings. In this country, we all have the luxury of being "worried well". We hear about illnesses like celiac sprue or Lyme disease and because we have some of the symptoms (medical students are the worst for contracting these "diseases"). We automatically worry that we may have the disease. These cases have undoubtedly been a challenging part of medicine. There has always been the complicated diabetics, hypertensives, atherosclerotics who seem to require more and more medicine while continuing to get sicker and sicker.

I am delighted to be able to present a new spectrum of possibilities to patients. I used to cringe when I had a patient come in and say "Doc, I'm tired. I have no energy. I get short of breath walking up the stairs, and by the way, my back, knees, and feet hurt." If these patients had seen doctors previously, they are generally on a bunch of meds causing undesirable side effects.

Now don't get me wrong, I respect what medicines can do for an individual, when all things are considered and the patient is invested in his/her own health. I ask patients HOW they are invested in their health. Are they exercising? What type of nutrition are they enjoying?

Have they considered how lack of sleep or too much stress is playing in their lives? Are they mindful of their environment and how it may affect them?

Low and behold, the savings account/investment portfolio in their WELL'TH looks deficient. I cannot emphasize this enough; healthcare reform starts with us, right now. Read this book, possibly others. Embrace and begin your journey towards wellness, and you will not be sorry.

According to the American Medical Society (AMA), exercise is medicine; free medicine that is available to everyone, everywhere. Countless studies support the role of exercise in the prevention of heart disease, hypertension, diabetes, dementia, certain cancers, depression, anxiety, asthma and erectile dysfunction. Several European nations have it right. The Swedish National Institute of Public Health helped prepare a 621 page book "Physical Activity in the Prevention and Treatment of Disease", with an emphasis on the remarkable benefits of exercise.

Here's how to incorporate exercise into your life. First off, realize where you are in the stages of change. Are you pre-contemplating, contemplating, planning, activating, or maintaining a healthy exercise lifestyle? Knowing this will help you get to the next step on the road to wellness. Don't rush. Take your time and ensure success. The last thing your body wants is you rushing into an exercise regimen for a month or two before losing interest, getting bored, or remembering that you don't like sweating.

Ultimately, exercise needs to be embraced as part of your new self, an investment in your well'th. It's not about getting into that new dress, looking good at your next school reunion, a New Year's resolution, or impressing a special someone. As Dr. Michael Roizen and Dr. Oz would say, it's about "you, you, you"! Now, if these things get you motivated and are short term goals toward the longer goal of health, then by all means focus. What I am getting at here is this; get started for the right reason, your "well'th".

Know thyself. Do you like working out with a reliable friend, or do you need the structure of a class? Would you enjoy competing in a race for the purpose of raising money for charity? What motivates you? What keeps you motivated? Write a list of Why's (for your health, your weight, your children, your spouse, etc.) Also prepare another list, of excuses, of why nots, and try to find answers to – hate to sweat, no time, etc. I believe that for your good health's sake, there is no time not to exercise. All of us should find the time during busy days for short exercise sessions. Consider walking during lunch.

Place your lists at the center of your refrigerator to stare at you and become motivators. Once in the planning stage, consider an exercise prescription in cooperation with your health care provider. Exercise prescriptions go by the mnemonic, 'FITT'. This stands for Frequency, Intensity, Type, and Time. Depending on where you are in your fitness, or what type of medical condition you have (fibromyalgia, chronic fatigue, etc.) will depend on where you start and how gradually you build. Ultimately you want to strive toward a goal. An example of a FITT prescription follows:

Frequency:	Start 2–3× per week
	Goal 4–6× per week
Intensity:	Start 60–70% of your MHR*
	Goal 65–85% of your MHR*
Type:	Both aerobic (on all exercise days), and resistance (2–3× per week)
Time:	Start 3–10 minutes
	Goal 30–60 minutes

(*MHR – Maximum Heart Rate generally defined as 220 – Age. So if you are 50 years old, your starting goal heart rate would be: (220–50) × 0.60 to 0.70 = 102–119 beats per minute.)

Build frequency and time first, by 10–20% per week until you have reached your goal, then build intensity. This is more likely to limit your risk of having a cardiac event or musculoskeletal injury. Remember there are different forms of aerobic and resistance exercises that can keep you in the game despite an injury or other setback.

Exercise to protect your "highways" (arteries) and ensure that your "car" (healthy HDL rather than Lethal LDL cholesterol) and engine (your heart and psyche) are high quality and in good working condition. Exercise so that the infrastructure, your bones and muscles, is not weak.

Still more is required for WELL'TH. Eight keys to wellness need to become part of your life for you to expect better health. Besides exercise, there is nutrition, stress management, sleep, mind activity, environment, spirituality, and health maintenance.

Nutrition is intimately bound to exercise. Ask any professional athlete. It makes sense that if you are exercising (actually even if you're not) and breaking down tissue, you would want to rebuild it with goodness. Let's not forget the phrase "you are what you eat". So even doing a great job with exercise, but consuming too many saturated fats (butter, animal fat) and refined sugars, chances are you are not as healthy as you could be, not to mention the incredible benefits found in vegetables and unhealthy food options.

So we know exercise and nutrition are good for you and possibly healing for what ails you. But what about sleep, stress? Certain hormones in your body are negatively affected by inadequate or too much sleep, as well as uncontrolled stress. Become mindful of these aspects of your health and how they play a role in your overall health.

Physicians daily see patients with chest pain, abdominal pain, eczema, depression, obesity, who are unaware, or not accepting of the impact of two wellness "keys" (sleep and stress) on their lives.

If you have made positive changes, reward yourself and keep moving toward a more positive, healthier self. Incorporating the analogy of the servicing your car, you cannot ignore a defective spark plug or timing belt just because you replaced the oil filter and pumped up the tires.

A patient of mine, despite being in his 40s with a couple stents and severe Coronary Artery Disease became hostile when I suggested that the three Mountain Dews, ½ pack of cigarettes, lack of exercise and insufficient sleep he was getting needed to change. He wanted me to realize he used to smoke two packs, drink alcohol, and use cocaine. Well yes, he made some impressive changes, but unfortunately missed the bigger picture of what could extend his life.

So be mindful of all the wellness keys, and invest in your Well'th. Consider this from the National Weight Loss Registry, an organization keeping track of folks who have been successful in losing weight and keeping it off.

Ninety-eight percent of registry participants report that they modified their food intake in some way to lose weight. Ninety-four percent increased physical activity with walking being the most frequently reported activity. Members kept weight off in several ways. Most maintain a low calorie, low fat diet and high levels of physical activity. Seventy-eight percent eat breakfast every day. Seventy-five percent weigh themselves at least once a week. Sixty-two percent watch less than ten hours of TV per week. Ninety percent exercise about an hour per day.

How you get there is unimportant. What's important is the end point of wellness and health. Focus on the "whys", not the "why not".

Dr. Katz practices sport and family medicine in Longmont, CO.

FAT FIGHTING AT ITS BEST:

Start a blog.
Get a dog.
Take a class.
Move your ass.
Don't just talk, walk the walk.
Cut harmful additives and sugar.
For natural fruits and a veggie burger.
Bad food has made you fat.
Good food will bring you back.
Wrong food has made you depressed.
Right food will make you feel your best.
Blessed with new positive energy.
You can exercise and become happy.
So throw out the cupcakes and Twinkies^{TM}.
And ride a bike while you watch TV.

—Wes Bagby

The power of why

To be and remain thin, we need to exercise and move about a lot more every day. Find an exercise you can do twice daily for at least 30 minutes per session. You can mix and match exercises and can break sessions into as many as you like. Within a few weeks, you'll feel healthier inside, and look better on the outside.

Think of exercise as a safe medicine that can improve your opinion of yourself. Once you put it to that test, you will find that exercising into better health is far better than anything you can buy at the drugstore or find in your medicine cabinet.

Exercising isn't easy. If it were, everyone would have perfect bodies. If eating properly and exercising were simple, heart disease would not be the nation's number one death maker. The fact is that starting an exercise program is unpleasant and difficult. Celebrities do not maintain their thin appearance because they love to exercise. They pay millions every year for fitness professionals to motivate them.

Whether you are famous or infamous, the hardest part about exercising is generating the motivation to stick with it. What you need are some secrets that offer you staying power. These are the "power of why".

> *The only exercise some people get is jumping to conclusions,*
> *running down their friends, side-stepping responsibility,*
> *and pushing their luck.*
>
> —Unknown

Mother Nature's 401K plan

Let's say you are walking along the beach and you find a bottle in the sand. Let's say a genie appeared out of the bottle and offers you the best 2 for 1 deal you can imagine. Two hours would be added to your life for every hour of exercise you complete. As much as you hate to exercise, would you refuse this offer?

Well, the genie's deal is for real. According to the American Heart Association, you can take advantage of this magical 2 for 1 deal anytime, no beach and no genie required. But it doesn't stop at adding years onto your life. In this deal you also will receive a higher quality of life during your remaining years. Think of it as Mother Nature's 401k plan for your life. For every hour of exercise, she not only gives you matching funds, but doubles them. And then she sweetens the deal. You get a better life with fewer hospital stays, less stress on you and your family, and more enjoyment.

What's the use of living longer if we can't be in shape for the ones we love? Exercise is the remedy for not only living longer, but carrying around an improved physical and mental outlook, a more enjoyable sex life, and not being a burden to others. Think about it this way; a longer, productive life with more joy, or a shorter life with more illness.

When you do, the temporary discomfort of beginning an exercise program looks ok. It's really not about whether you have time to exercise, but how much your loved ones will miss you if you don't.

Here's your choice. Exercise every day, or get sick and need an operation from someone you don't know, or more importantly, who doesn't know you. Assuming you recover from the operation, guess what you will be told before leaving the hospital and filling your new prescriptions; that you need to begin an exercise program! So, you can start exercising after a heart attack or you can start now. You're intelligent. Start now.

Reasons to exercise: A third of American adults have heart problems. The rate skyrockets to over 70 percent after the age of 60. Being obese or even overweight reduces life spans. Six out of 10 Americans are overweight or obese, so you are not alone. But who wants to be a member of a society of fatness?

In addition to weight control, exercise helps to reverse heart disease. It helps control cholesterol levels and diabetes. It slows bone loss associated with advancing age, lowers the risk of certain cancers, and reduces anxiety.

Fewer than one in three Americans exercise regularly at healthful levels, and nearly two-thirds of them are overweight or obese. See the connection? A difference one can of soda a day (150 calories) or 60 minutes of brisk daily walking can add or subtract 15 pounds to your weight each year. Just imagine if you eliminated sugared soda and decided to walk about an hour a day. You would double your results and lose 30 pounds in a year. Knowing this, can you really ever say again with a straight face that Coke™ is "it"?

Think of exercise as food to realize what you are burning off. One hour of walking burns off the calorie equivalent of a typical jelly filled doughnut (300 calories). You can also do the reverse and think of food as exercise. Before you stop at the drive-thru on your way home from work, consider that a double cheeseburger with fries and soft drink is equivalent to 2.5 hours of running at a 10 minute per mile pace. If you're committed to getting thin, which is easier, driving past the drive thru and going home for a nutritious vegetable soup, or running 2.5 hours? I haven't seen any restaurant make a double cheeseburger that good.

To be thin, exercising is essential whether it's dancing, swimming, jogging, biking, hiking, gardening, yoga, Tai chi. This chapter focuses on two helpful exercises; walking, the easiest, and sex, the one that's more fun.

Walk more, live longer

Anywhere is walking distance if you've got the time.
—Stephen Wright

Being entirely honest with oneself is a good exercise.
—Sigmund Freud

My idea of exercise is a good brisk sit.
—Phyllis Diller

Another good reducing exercise consists in placing both hands against the table edge and pushing back.
—Robert Quillen

Take brisk walks or don't bother. Walk for an hour or more a day. Walk as if you're in a hurry to be somewhere else. The number of daily walks you take doesn't matter. It's the total walking time that counts. Once walking becomes routine, mix some slow jogging into it, especially down hills. This will get your heart pumping more, providing additional benefits.

Besides helping you lose weight, walking adds to your overall well being. Here are reasons for lots of walking: Walking is good for the brain. Women who walk more have better brain function than those who walk less. Walking is good for bones. Walkers have higher leg bone density than non-walkers. Walking strengthens the heart and cuts the risk of heart attack. Walkers live longer than non-walkers.

Mindful walking helps remove mental clutter and chatter. While walking, focus on the beauty of your natural surroundings or the many positives in your life (the ability to walk being a big one). Count the trees and bushes you walk by, note the animals you happen upon. Listen to sounds you don't get to hear while cooped up at work all day. Maybe you hear nothing at all. In that case, enjoy the silence while you walk your way to a more healthy you. When you get home, enjoy a cup of peppermint tea.

Walking with a friend makes the experience more enjoyable. Time goes by faster, but walking alone is better than not walking at all. Most of us know that walking is great for legs, heart, butt, and other parts, but did you know walking also can flatten bellies? After 14 weeks of brisk walking, women in one study shrunk belly fat by 20 percent without cutting back on their eating. The longer the walks, the better your health, the thinner your body.

> *A vigorous five-mile walk will do more good than all the medicine and psychology in the world.*
> —White House doctor Carl Dudley White, MD

Bedroom workouts

> *Don't have sex man. It leads to kissing and pretty soon you have to start talking to them.*
> —Steve Martin

I'm at an age when food has taken the place of sex in my life. In fact, I've just had a mirror put over my kitchen table.

—Rodney Dangerfield

When I'm good, I'm very, very good, but when I'm bad I'm better.

—Mae West

Exercise and balanced eating can revive a dormant sex drive. Sex produces feel-good chemicals in the brain. It satisfies parts of the brain that sends signals tempting us to eat unhealthy food. When you lose weight, your sex drive increases and the quality of sex improves. Here's how to restore sexual energy:

Lose weight. Losing even ten pounds may stimulate sex hormones. Replace harmful foods with nutritious ones. Engage in exercise that generates blood flow to the pelvic area. Renew intimacy with someone special. Exercising in bed is a great way to keep fit. Active women produce more estrogen and have shinier hair. Men over 60 who engage in sex live longer than men who don't. Thanks to sweating, skin pores are cleansed. People feel and look younger from healthy sex. They are happier, better rested, and more content with their lives.

One expert in bedroom exercise (a housewife) wrote: "I recommend having sex five times a week since it's free and a lot of fun. Making love is my favorite form of exercise." Keep in mind that what you give in bed is likely what's coming back to you. Be playfully creative. Become the self-assured lover your bed partner desires. Good sex is about intimacy; physical, emotional, conversational. Mental lovemaking counts even more than having the right touch. Say something loving and sexy to your partner and mean it. You know what she/he wants to hear. Talk the right talk. Otherwise what's the point?

When we get too little love, we may compensate by overeating. We seek satisfaction in food in a vain attempt to replace the love/sex we really need. This is the connection between love-making and getting thin. When we get thinner, the sex gets better. When the sex is good, we want more of it, and less food. Why? Because we want to have more energy for more sex. Overeating tires us out.

So find somebody to love. Interest your partner in the sexual you and fall in love all over again. Replacing excess weight with love is a terrific exchange. Like brisk walking, good sex should be a frequent activity. Let it become a healthful, beautiful addiction that helps you keep your fingers out of the cookie jar.

Exercise caution: The (positive) stress of vigorous sex late in life can be dangerous, even life threatening. Do not leap right into it from a sedentary lifestyle. Get into shape or you run a higher risk having a heart attack during sex. Like other exercising, it takes time to achieve a healthy level of fitness where you can vigorously and safely enjoy a thrilling bedroom romp with nothing but naughtiness on your mind. Have a medical somebody examine you. If ok, get it on.

It's not true I had nothing on, I had the radio on.

—Marilyn Monroe

Dancing queen

by Allison Kummery

I've never had a weight issue, sorry, hate me all you want, but it's true. I was active, had older siblings who kept me on the run constantly, and got bored staying in one place for too long. I grew up in a middle class family. We never ate out because with four kids we just couldn't plain afford to. My mother cared enough about our health to save us from the likes of fast food dinners. She painstakingly made us home cooked meals until the time I left the house to attend college. Sure, I had the rare happy meal from time to time, but for the most part, healthy eating was instilled in me through my upbringing.

Only once in my life did I come to a crossroads when the battle of the bulge came into play, and it happened right after my freshman year in college. That's right, even thin, energetic me, was too weak to defeat the "freshman 15". I'm sure some of you are thinking: "I wish I was only 15 pounds overweight." I never noticed it coming on, but then the day arrived when my favorite jeans would no longer button. Unfortunately I was too bogged down with school to make a weight loss effort so my freshman 15 turned into my sophomore 60.

So I did what any fat little sophomore girl would do and I changed my major to exercise. What a quick fix! You only realize just how out of shape you are when you step out of your humdrum comfort zone and really shake things up. The capability of our bodies to adapt is amazing.

I started teaching ballroom dancing after college. I was not formally trained, but dancing came naturally, and with practice and patience from kind dance partners, I learned. Not only did I learn, but I lost a lot of weight, and made a lot of money, and had a fantastic time doing it. This is the stuff dreams are made of. I'd like you to consider dance as one of the forms of exercise you use to lose weight and be healthier. Here's why:

Dancing is easy and can be done anywhere with or without music, with or without clothes, with or without equipment/props. It's simple. There needn't be a celebration or a special event.

Dancing can be an emotional connection between two human beings. You may not have a lover and enjoy the five day a week sex plan earlier described by an anonymous housewife, but you can find a dance partner. It's been proven that couples who dance together have fewer arguments than couples who do not. The mere act of looking into one another's eyes while touching in a simple dance hold actually promotes the release of serotonin from the brain. Thus the thought pattern, "I like this guy. Dancing with him is fun, and we should do this more often. He makes me happy".

It doesn't have to be a romantic connection between dance partners. It can be a friend, family member, or a stranger in which the connection shared is one of pure joy. I've never seen someone dance angry. Not only that, but if you dance a lot and get really good, you can bring great joy to others. They watch you dance and become moved at the beauty you bring.

Dancing is not only good for the soul, it's profoundly efficient at burning calories and strengthening the body on a physical level. The movements of dance are unrestrained and uninhibited by fitness equipment or devices, allowing your body to move in ways comfortable to its own make up and rhythms. It improves core strength effectively because most people have a tendency to flail their legs and arms while dancing, thus creating a stabilizing reaction throughout the abdomen and back. People also enjoy thrusting and gyrating moves, good for increasing core strength. Beyond the physical is the mental. Learning steps to a dance can be compared to doing a crossword puzzle. You are forcing the brain to think in new patterns and create new neural pathways. Your coordination and balance improve. Your body remembers how to shift and counterbalance through the movements you learned.

Did I mention it's fun? To determine if something is good for you, I refer to the components of true wellness being spiritual, intellectual, psychological, physical, emotional, social, and occupational. When these elements are balanced in your life, I would describe you as "happy". Here is how dance helps attain wellness through these components.

SPIRITUAL: A woman once told me that she was on a cruise and did not have a partner to dance with so she said a silent prayer and asked God to dance with her. She recounted the experience as if she was describing being saved. She had never felt God's presence so strongly nor danced with such passion in her life. It was a joyful time she shared with the Almighty. Beyond this woman's account are hundreds of cultures and tribes that use dance as a traditional form of worship.

PSYCHOLOGICAL: Dance produces feelings of wellness on a chemical level. Promoting the release and uptake of serotonin, a natural mood booster, is a happy little side effect of shaking your tail feather. Why take LSD or Prozac to feel good when you can dance. Intellectually, people sense you're smart when you dance. Of course you can be a box of rocks, but chances are if you've taken the initiative to learn a few moves, there's something to be said for your IQ.

PHYSICAL: This goes without saying really. You work absolutely every inch of your body when you dance from your toes to the tips of your fingers. Dancing increases metabolic burn, circulatory flow, respiratory strength, endurance, balance, coordination, and overall muscle tone. With movement and increased circulation, joints are exercised and vital synovial fluid replenished, keeping joints supple and nourished.

EMOTIONAL: Benefits of dance come from within or can be shared with another producing positive, wide ranging emotions. Picture a father dancing with his only daughter on the day of her wedding, getting ready to release her into the arms of a man he hopes will care and provide for her. Picture a budding young love dancing at the prom. Or a ballerina floating across the stage with the utmost elegance and poise. Picture yourself listening to your favorite song in a car that's stuck in traffic. Note the desire to stop the car and dance to the melody.

SOCIAL: The social aspects of dancing are obvious. Most parties or social events have a band, a dance floor, or a Congo line. It's almost harder not to dance than it is to actually get in on the action. Don't be shy! Grab someone or just go it alone and dance like no one is watching.

Night clubs offer dancing to Latin music, country music, big band, rock and roll, hip hop, jazz. Pick one and get a group of girl friends to go out dancing, and celebrate your friendships with one another.

OCCUPATIONAL: Well, maybe this doesn't apply to everyone, but since I'm a dance teacher I guess I've got it made. But if your office plays music, you can dance and blame it on them. Tell them I said so. Happy dancing. Turn up the volume and trim down your waist.

Allison Kummery's photo is on the front cover. She teaches Zumba at Reflex Arts Dance & Yoga studio in Sarasota, FL.

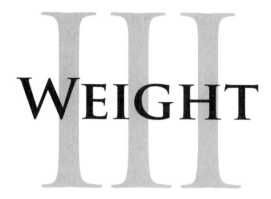

WEIGHT

Behavior Modification, or behaviorism is based on the proposition that just about everything we do (thinking, sleeping, feeling, learning, eating) is behavior.

Business uses the science of human behavior to "hook us" into buying products, good and bad, time after time. Many expand our waistlines and harm our health.

"Good" behavioral guidelines in this book teach you how to "escape" from "bad", addictive, harmful, toxic garbage on grocer shelves. Understanding something about behavioral science can help you create a healthful lifestyle with more vigor, more happiness, and less weight.

Healthy brain, slender body

When brains work well, other body parts work better too. America's top brain expert, Daniel Amen, MD, addresses this in his book

"Change Your Brain, Change Your Body." Amen concludes that brains, like other body parts, can become imbalanced and require treatment. Corrective treatments include vitamin supplements, healing foods, positive thinking, and more. According to Amen, various brain disorders can keep people overweight, or lead to binge-eating and sickness. Bear in mind that each person's brain is unique. There is no single cure-all that fits everyone.

Consuming addictive foods or over-exposure to chemicals are factors in some brain disorders. As much as possible, we need to keep toxins out of our bodies and eat properly. An excess of salty, sugary foods can be harmful to brain, heart and body. Overeating can become addictive, leading to memory loss and emotional disarray. Prevention can be found through eating healthful foods. Suggestions for keeping brains healthy follow:

- Eat a balanced diet. Brains need a limited number of calories. A thin brain is a happy brain.
- Drink plenty of pure water. Your brain consists of over 65% water. Dehydration damages brain cells.
- Eat wild fish caught in cold ocean waters, especially salmon.
- Walk daily. Walking keeps brains younger.
- Rapid motion exercises such as ping pong and dancing increase blood flow to the brain. More oxygen and nutrients lead to better processing of complex thoughts.
- Berries and other fruit are good for brains.
- Beans, chickpeas and walnuts are good brain foods.
- Puzzles and mind exercises strengthen brains.
- Ten minute naps refresh the mind & improve memory.
- A daily multiple vitamin may improve memory and mood.
- Reduce caffeine intake. Caffeine reduces blood flow, depriving brain cells of nutrients.

- Don't smoke or hang around others when they are smoking. Brains and nicotine don't mix well.

- Reduce stress. It is associated with memory loss. Meditate. Hang out with positive people as one good way to keep calm.

- Know that the freedom of good health lies in the ability to maintain a positive relationship with health enhancing foods. Start a healthy food revolution within yourself today.

How to lose weight

You may be reading this book because you intend to lose weight. Perhaps you want to be more attractive, have more energy, live longer, or improve your love life. An array of solutions are here to help you get thin. You know yourself better than anyone else knows you, so use whatever works for you. Taking good care of yourself goes hand in hand with health and happiness. A thin you likely will live a longer and healthier life than an overweight you. Intuitively we know this, so then why carry around too much weight in the first place? Here are reasons:

- We got addicted to fattening, salty, sugary foods.
- We overeat because we can't stop eating.
- We need to learn a new healthier way of life.
- We tend to be couch potatoes.
- We wrongly think being overweight is our fate because obesity runs in the family. The good news is we can change. We can eat in a way that will help achieve the right weight. We can make better choices for ourselves. If millions of smokers can quit a bad tobacco addiction, and they have, we can stop overeating and can keep harmful foods out of our bodies.

When we eat healthy, we become healthy. We look younger and feel better. Taking responsibility for our diet and exercise routines can lead to a longer, healthier life. Natural, fiber rich foods are satisfying, and less likely to be overeaten. Embrace quality over quantity. The ability to eat modest portions of high quality foods may not happen right away, so be patient. Portion control can be learned.

Choosing healthful foods is the first step. To make weight loss permanent, creating a new way of eating is called for, a new, permanent lifestyle that contains mindful, healthful eating at its core.

The next step is to begin making changes in your lifestyle. Start small and find ways to fill your days with movement. Be active whenever you have the chance. Stretch, twist, swing your arms, move your legs, dance, practice Yoga or Tai Chi. Turn the TV off, unglue yourself from the computer and move your body. Find stairs and climb them. Whenever possible, ride your bike or walk. It might take longer to get where you're going, but you will get thin a lot faster. You can walk yourself thin! Brisk walks tone the stomach, curb appetites, and burn calories.

Small portions of healthy foods plus lots of movement equal a thin, healthy you. Becoming mindful of eating habits lets you enjoy the good things in life; leaner body, better health, more energy. You can create a new, thin you by loving and taking better care of yourself. Your brain and body will return the favor. Welcome to the first phase of being thin.

The doctor of the future will give us no medication, but will interest his patients in the care of the human frame, diet, and in the cause and prevention of disease.

—Thomas Edison

Weight loss strategies

This book adopts principles developed by experts in the science of human behavior. Over the years these methods have helped people end smoking addiction, treat mental illness, and control weight. Behavior

modification can be self taught by identit
monitoring your behavior, and finally, chan;
produced the problem. Replacing undesirabl
healthy eating behaviors lead to desirable weig

The first step is to get a clear picture of wh
you eat, and when you eat. Behavior modificati   ......s to
the reasons why people overeat. With increased awareness, you will
connect with the wisdom of eating smaller food portions. You will
find ways to make good health maintenance part of your lifestyle.
Consider the following weight loss strategies:

Establish a weight target and stick to it. Suppose you intend
to lose 30 pounds. Do so by losing 1–2 pounds a week. Slow and
steady weight loss is the safest combination. Part of achieving your
weight objective is keeping your mind focused on it every day. Dieting cannot be an on-again, off-again affair. This is where developing
a dietary lifestyle comes into play. If you only change your eating
habits while you're dieting, it's likely that you will join the 90 percent
of dieters who quickly regain weight after leaving the diet.

If you fail to plan, you plan to fail.

—Proverb

Keep a daily food journal. Keep accurate records of everything
you eat for the next two weeks. Everything that's food related should
go into your journal. Note the times for meals and snacks. A food
journal helps to identify all the foods you are eating and why. Note in
your journal any unusual aspect of your eating. Did you snack when
tired, bored or angry? Did you notice a "worst" food time, or any
specific times or occasions when you ate too much? Were you okay
with portion sizes? Did you have binges or eat unhealthy foods? As
you review the week, consider what caused overeating.

Write a menu of foods that you intend to eat the following
day. Include everything, even snacks and water. Design menus with

al of being thin and healthy in mind. Food choices should be
ritious, filling, and of moderate portion sizes. When you finish
your list, set a personal resolve to strictly follow the menu plan.
Create menus at times when you are not hungry. Suggestions for
food menus are listed at the back of this book.

Weigh yourself once a week at same time of day and record it.
After a week of record keeping and sticking to your food menus,
evaluate your progress.

Weighing less each week will make you feel good about your
progress. Gaining weight, or being stuck on a plateau means you
need to make adjustments.

Dieters who weigh themselves regularly lose more weight than
those who don't. Weighing motivates us to take additional steps
when necessary, such as exercising more and eating less. Remember
though, a scale is just a tool. Don't let it rule your life, affect your
feelings, or thwart your progress. Harsh numbers on a scale must not
defeat your sense of self worth. Next week you'll weigh less.

If you feel too hungry, add proteins to your diet, such as
hummus, fish, hard-boiled egg whites, skinless baked chicken. Dr.
Louis Arrone, an internationally recognized diet and obesity expert, explains that eating healthy, high protein foods early in the
day can lead to feeling full much longer than otherwise. Foods
containing lots of protein provide nourishment and eliminate
hunger pangs.

Eat slowly. It's important that you take your time because your
stomach needs 20 minutes to tell your brain that it is full. Put your
fork down to slow down between bites. Keep your eyes on the prize
by visualizing a thin you.

FASTING can be your winning ticket to weight loss. One
type of fast involves eating fruit and water for 36 hours, beginning at
6 p.m. on the first day. Drink more water than usual and snack on
fresh fruit. Don't go for more than five hours without eating. While
results may vary, expect to lose 2–3 pounds each time you do this fast.

You may feel less hungry after the fast than when you started 36 hours earlier. Fasting curbs appetites by shrinking the size of the stomach.

GET PAID to lose weight! Here's a benefit to belonging to a weight loss group. You and friends create a pool of money each month, say $10 each. Everyone weighs themselves simultaneously at the beginning and ending of the month. The two people who lose the most weight in the 30 days share the total amount in the kitty. It's fun and simple and highly motivating to establish and maintain a "thin" lifestyle.

Reward yourself in various ways. Pat yourself on the back each day you stick to your diet. Create a reward system by making a check mark in your food journal each day that you eat well. When you earn seven checks in a row give yourself a small gift, like a trip to the movies, a new magazine, or a rose. Or save the check marks for a month and treat yourself to something a little more lavish, like a massage, a new piece of clothing, or a night on the town. You may even want to treat yourself to a food item not on your diet, like dark chocolate or cheeseburger. Food rewards should be limited to one every three or four weeks.

Sleep well. Give your body quality sleep time. Finish eating a few hours before your bed time. Night-time eaters weigh about eight percent more than people who eat all their food during the day.

Other weight loss ideas: Keep the refrigerator stocked with nutritious food only. Make cut up raw fruits and veggies available for easy snacking. Drink lots of water as a sure fire way to feel full. Always eat breakfast, even if it's just toast and tea. Take the time to read labels. Choose food wisely and remain mindful, even vigilant about protecting your right to eat properly.

> *When hungry I eat, when tired I sleep. Fools laugh at me.*
> *The wise understand.*
> —Zen Master Rinzai

My advice if you insist on slimming: Eat as much as you like, just don't swallow it.

—Harry Secombe

Don't dig your grave with a knife and a fork.

—Proverb

Mindfulness

Do you taste your food before swallowing it? I mean really taste it for flavor, chewiness, freshness, enjoyment. Or is mealtime simply a food inhaling experience when you think about everything besides the food you're eating? Mindful eating can help with weight control, and recognizing when enough food eaten really is enough.

When we focus on food in all of its aspects, purchase, preparation, consumption, we make wise food choices and feel healthier. Mindfulness improves our decision-making abilities and peace of mind. Patients suffering from anxiety, depression and eating disorders often learn mindfulness as part of their treatment. Being selective about the foods you buy, the way you prepare food, when you eat, and how much you eat, all help to make you thin.

Consider the influences on your food selections. TV commercials are designed to sell you stuff, good and bad. So are displays at grocery stores. As you walk about the store, ask yourself, "do I really need this"? Consider how foods you consider buying will make you feel. Avoid buying what's harmful to your body, your mind, your wallet.

Making mindful food decisions when you're hungry isn't easy. So shop and prepare meals before the level of hunger rises. Doing so will help you to focus on what's really important – choosing the right foods, eating slowly, chewing well. Consider the way your food is prepared; baked, fried, raw or steamed. Notice the smells, taste, quality, freshness and texture. When your thoughts wander away from the food experience, gently invite your mind back into focus. Reflect again on how the food you are buying, preparing or eating will make you feel.

This is all a lot to chew on, but with practice you can eat mindfully. This is one form of personal discipline that can lead to a better all around life management. One way to stay focused on the practice of eating is to count the number of times you chew each bite of food. Another method is to notice the way it feels to chew your food. Observe the colors of your food – the brighter the natural color, the healthier. Think of purple berries, green spinach, golden sweet potatoes. Smell the food you're eating. Take time to enjoy what soon will become yourself.

A display of appreciation is indicated within the practice of mindful eating. Before your meal, pause to offer silent or spoken thanks for the gift of healthy food. With a little practice, mindfulness can lead all to a healthy, thin life.

Solutions to weighty problems

The Problem: BINGES

Solutions: Keep binge foods out of the house, and have fruits and veggies on hand. When eaten slowly, half a bagel with drops of olive oil will turn off the urge to binge. So does a ripe banana. Drink a glass of water and try to relax. The urge to binge fades in less than a minute.

Find something constructive to do. Join a dance group that meets after work. Go to the gym. Mind-body practices like Yoga and Tai Chi can help counteract binging. Besides improving your body's flexibility and strength, yoga will make you more sensitive to your food choices. Yoga empowers you to listen to your body's messages. With practice, you can tune into your appetite and become a better eater.

The Problem: PLATEAU (Stuck on too much weight)

Solutions: For another week, record everything you eat. Create new "thin" menus consisting of smaller portions. Identify problems that caused you to stop losing weight. Remove high calorie foods from your house. Walk more and watch less TV. Leave the table before your feel "full." Feeling full from eating means you already ate too much. It makes you feel tired. Experiment with ways to cut back on portion sizes.

The Problem: FEELING ALONE

Solutions: Explain your weight goal to your friends and family, and invite them to get involved with your diet. Loved ones will also benefit from healthy eating awareness. If support isn't forthcoming, make some new friends. Join a diet group. Losing weight with friends is more effective than dieting alone. Explore ways to help others. Volunteer at your local library or animal shelter. Stacking books and walking dogs are good exercise options.

The Problem: ANGER

Solutions: Use humor to cool your anger. Enjoy a funny movie, read silly stories, or watch the comedy channel. How easy is it to be angry when you're laughing at life's absurdities? Yoga, meditation and exercise all help with anger management.

The Problem: FATIGUE

Solutions: Practice counting your breaths as a way to fall asleep. Getting enough sleep prevents your body from storing fat. Lack of sleep increases cravings for fattening foods. Go to bed when you're tired and aim to sleep for eight hours.

The Problem: OVEREATING

Solutions: Drink water 20 minutes before meals. Chew your food thoroughly and slowly. Put your fork down between bites. Fast eaters are three times as likely to be overweight than slow eaters. Moderate your portion sizes: Use a salad plate instead of a dinner plate to make it seem like there's more food in front of you. Choose "thin" and nutritious foods like corn tortillas instead of bread; fresh fruit instead of fruit pastries. By eating healthy, whole foods, your body will need less food to feel satisfied.

The Problem: STRESS

Solutions: Exercise! Walk, dance, swim, bike, hike. Exercise your mind by painting, reading, writing, bird watching, solving puzzles. Meditate and practice yoga. Listen to music. Avoid stress-inducing foods containing processed sugar. Smile and laugh. Buy and enjoy foods that are healing.

To enhance health, we need to think outside the Devil's food cake and chocolate chip cookie boxes. For the sake of those you love, let a healthy food revolution begin first in your own mind. Menus for speedy weight loss are at the back of the book.

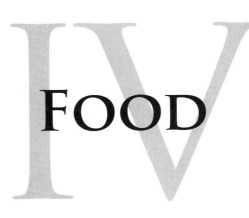

FOOD

Tell me what you eat, and
I will tell you what you are.

—Antheime Brillat-Savarin

It's not what you're eating, it's what's eating you.

—Unknown

YOU better cut the pizza in four pieces because
I'm not hungry enough to eat six.

—Yogi Berra

The devil came to me last night and asked what
I wanted in exchange for my soul. I still can't believe
I said pizza. Friggin' cravings.

—Marc Ostroff

Some say healthy eating is unaffordable. False! At the end of the day, the cost of apples and oranges is a lot less than the cost of open heart surgery. The old saying, quality not quantity, can be applied nicely here. Keeping to modest portions of high quality foods permanently to be thin permanently doesn't happen automatically. You need to take charge of yourself, walk a lot more, eat perhaps a lot less. It's up to you; a longer, healthier life or one shortened by continuing to obey food cravings that are bad for your waistline and health.

Rules of eating: Don't buy foods containing more than four or five ingredients. If a food company needs to jack up products with chemicals you can't pronounce, it's not for you. "If it don't rot, it should not be bought." Imagine the damage foods kept chemically "fresh" can do when they enter your gut, liver, heart and brain. Leave such foods on store shelves.

Enjoy meals with people you care about. It's a time for bonding with those who enjoy the company of one another. Buy foods favored by your great grandparents. The 1900 generation had health problems, but those folks didn't suffer epidemics that ravage 2011 America, diabetes, cancer, heart disease, obesity. Consider several meatless days a week, or go meatless altogether. That alone may extend your life by making you healthier.

Buy foods that don't add salt or sugar. Limit the food on your plate to three items or fewer. We eat less when less food is in front of us. Share dessert. You'll capture the flavor and miss half the calories. If your dessert happens to be pie (it shouldn't be), eat the filling and skip the crust.

Leave the table feeling a little hungry. You'll enjoy more energy. Substitute high calorie breakfast foods like granola with low calorie cereals like shredded wheat. You get just as full on fewer calories.

When diet is wrong, medicine is of no use.
When diet is correct, medicine is of no need.

—Proverb

Super foods

When you consider the undesirable health consequences of addictive foods, their appeal begins to fade. For a thin, healthy future, consider these nourishing food choices. Some can help make a thin you and also contain the power to heal.

APPLE: This super fruit should be part of your daily diet. Apples help to curb your appetite and are cancer fighters. The fiber in apples expands in your stomach, making you feel full while drawing out bad cholesterol. Oxidants in apples help prevent prostrate and lung cancer, and may help slow the aging process. Low calorie apples fill you up without making you fill out. Enjoy apple wedges before meals to boost your weight loss efforts. The peel contains anticancer properties. Always wash an apple before eating.

AVOCADOS are a great substitute for butter, mayonnaise or cream cheese. They provide important vitamins, minerals, healthy fat and protein. Try adding slices to salads or soups. Enjoy avocados in moderation as they are high in calories.

BANANAS: This yellow fruit lowers high blood pressure and protects against heart disease. Caution: bananas are high in calories, so enjoy in moderation.

BLUEBERRIES: A nutritional powerhouse all by itself, blueberries go well with just about anything. Blueberries help reduce age related diseases and long-term memory loss.

BEANS & LENTILS are chock full of healthy nutrients. Think chickpeas, black beans and kidney beans. Lentils are first cousin of the bean and the pea. Lentils are protein rich, nutritious and affordable. Think lentil stew with lots of veggies. The Mediterranean diet is considered to be one healthiest approaches to eating, and lentils are a centerpiece of this menu. Fiber-rich lentils help protect the heart by lowering cholesterol and keeping blood sugar levels down.

I'm President of the United States and
I'm not going to eat any broccoli.

—George W. Bush Sr.

The belly is ungrateful. It always forgets
we already gave it something.

—Proverb

CABBAGE: The ancient Greeks and Romans believed that cabbage surpassed all other vegetables. An excellent source of fiber and vitamins. Cabbage soup will heal the coldest soul.

CAULIFLOWER can be eaten cooked, raw or pickled. It is nutritious, high in fiber, low in fat, and acts as a cancer fighter. Cauliflower is a good substitute for starchy potatoes.

COTTAGE CHEESE: If you include dairy in your diet, consider low-fat cottage cheese. High in protein, cottage cheese fills you up and keeps you satisfied for a long time. Try it with rye toast and apples. Recommended brand: 1% Friendship, with "no added salt" painted on the container.

DARK CHOCOLATE is a mixed blessing food. It's delicious and heart healthy when it contains at least 60% cacao. Small portions of dark chocolate increase brain blood flow and could make you smarter. Chocolate is high in sugar, fat and salt, so enjoy in moderation. Be sure to clean your teeth and gums after each chocolate experience to avoid a $1,600 root canal. Avoid milk chocolate altogether as there are zero health benefits.

EGG WHITES are a healthy, low calorie source of protein. Eating egg whites early in the day will help to curb your appetite. Prepare hard boiled eggs in advance for easy snacking.

FISH: Alaskan fish such as salmon, perch, and halibut are low in calories and high in protein. While more expensive, Alaskan fish is less polluted than other fish. Eating three or more servings a week will help make you healthy and thin. Wild salmon reduces blood pressure and the risk of having a heart attack. Other nutritious fish to consider are mackerel, herring and tuna.

GRAPES and their various forms (raisins, red wine) are cancer and heart disease fighters. Eating purple concord grapes will help to sharpen your mind.

HUMMUS tastes great and is good for you. Its smooth texture replaces mayonnaise and can be used as a meat substitute. This high protein food goes well with sliced cucumbers on salt free crackers. Try hummus on a flat bread tomato sandwich. Recommended brands: Sabra™ and Sam's Club. Both taste great.

NUTS are valued for their good taste and high nutritional value. Walnuts are loaded with omega-3 fatty acids that are good for hearts. Nuts are mood enhancers. People who eat nuts have fewer junk food cravings, and live two to three years longer than people who don't. Nuts are high in calories, so eat small quantities (approximately 10) of salt-free nuts for optimal health benefits.

OATMEAL lowers cholesterol and reduces the risk of heart disease. It's filling and tastes great with yogurt, cinnamon, raisins, blueberries and/or honey. Oatmeal is a perfect food choice any time of day.

An onion can make people cry, but there has never been a veggie invented to make them laugh.
—Will Rogers

Second opinion: Do not eat garlic or onions for their smell will reveal that you are a peasant.
—Cervantes

This cabbage, these potatoes, these carrots, these onions will soon become me. Such a tasty fact!
—Mike Garafalo

RICE and almond milk are delicious with shredded wheat and blueberries, and win out over the milk of any four-footed creature.

RYE is a grain bread that fills you up and also keeps your hunger at bay for many hours. Researchers found that two slices of rye toast in the morning will decrease hunger both before and after lunch. But do not buy "rye" bread that's not really rye. Most breads sold as "rye" contain more wheat than rye is the MAIN grain in the loaf. Don't be fooled by bread makers. Buy real rye. There's a difference.

SHREDDED WHEAT: Eating bite sized shredded wheat improves digestion. The fiber in wheat clears out digestive pipes and has a cleansing effect. If you feel an evening binge coming on, you can make it a healthful experience by enjoying a guilt-free bowl of shredded wheat, blueberries and/or raisins in rice milk.

SPINACH: Vitamin rich spinach gave Popeye his power plus his good looks. Because of spinach, Olive Oil's boy friend never got macular degeneration. Popeye's career ended with a strong heart and no obesity. Eat spinach as often as you like.

SWEET POTATOES & YAMS: One of the most nutritional foods, sweet potatoes are a veritable warehouse of vitamins and fiber. In 1920, Americans ate on average 31 pounds of sweet potatoes a year. Today, we eat an average of four pounds a year. Is the rise in cancer rates related to the quality of our food choices?

TOMATOES: What's a sandwich without slices, a pizza without tomato sauce, or a salad without the red color? Tomatoes are cancer fighters and help prevent heart disease.

VEGETABLE JUICE: Drink a glass of sodium-free veggie juice 20 minutes before lunch or dinner as a healthy way to curb your appetite. Adding grape juice improves the taste.

Soup offers many blessings. Eating low salt, low fat vegetable laden soup as your main meal will make you thin. Colorful veggies tossed into a pot of water or broth quickly turns into delicious, nourishing soup.

If it grows out of the ground or someone can pick it off a tree, chances are it's good for you.

—Unknown

Fruit winners: cherries, berries, plums, mango, dates, figs, oranges, prunes, cantaloupe, honeydew, strawberries, watermelon, peaches, pears. Buy locally grown produce whenever possible.

Veggie favorites: asparagus, cucumber, broccoli, peppers, eggplant, collard greens, Brussels sprouts, garlic, mushroom, pumpkin, beets, celery, zucchini, lettuce and carrots.

Mediterranean Health: The Mediterranean diet creates better mental health, reduces the risk of heart disease and lowers blood sugar. This diet emphasizes small portions of high quality foods such as veggies, fish, nuts, fruit, lentils and grains. Olive oil replaces butter and margarine.

Brain healthy foods

For optimal brain health, eat a diet that includes wild ocean fish, asparagus, Brussels sprouts, blueberries, whole grain cereals, and plenty of pure water. Celery fights off destructive inflammation of the brain's memory center. Artichokes protect blood vessels and help prevent the onset of strokes.

Mental agility foods: Turmeric in mustard activates genes that clean up our brains. Eggs contain selenium, slowing aging of the brain. Blueberries, spinach, kale, and collard greens also slow mental decline. Peppermint tea helps you focus, and boosts mental performance. Drivers are more alert and less anxious after drinking mint tea. Wild salmon and mackerel reduce forgetfulness, confusion and memory loss. Walnuts even look like a brain and give us an added mental boost. Nuts are good for reversing the effects of stress. Wheat germ also assists with stress reduction and increases physical endurance. Try a half a cup of wheat germ with yogurt or oatmeal.

Negative calorie foods: Some fruits and vegetables actually burn more calories in the digestion process than they contain. It seems absurd, but perhaps the more of these foods you eat, the more weight you lose. Negative calorie foods include apples, asparagus, beets, broccoli, cabbage, carrots, cauliflower, celery, cucumbers, grapefruit, lettuce, oranges, pineapples, raspberries, spinach, strawberries, turnips and zucchini. Enjoy.

Starchy foods: White bread, white potatoes and white rice all produce empty calories. Who needs that? Nourishing, high roughage, starchy foods such as multigrain cereals, sweet potatoes and brown rice will trigger a sense of fullness in both brain and belly. You can eat less of these foods and still feel full.

Belly fat fighting foods contain flavonoids that reduce belly bulge by increasing body metabolism. These waistline trimming foods include pears, apples, tea, onions, beans and sweet peppers.

Heart healthy foods

Unsalted nuts, beans, peas, asparagus, Brussels sprouts, broccoli, artichokes, cabbage, squash, carrots, greens, green beans, peas, pumpkin, mushrooms, onions, spinach, tomatoes, plums, berries, raisins, prunes, pineapples, melons, peaches, mangoes, oranges, grapes, cherries, dates, apples, bananas, pears, figs. Oatmeal and whole grain cereals with no sugar or salt added. Wild fish caught in cold ocean waters.

Acid and alkaline foods: Acidic foods weaken bones and muscles. Alkaline foods have an opposite effect. Acidic foods include alcohol, bread, beef, cereal, milk, nuts, rice and animal products such as cheese and eggs. Fruits and veggies are alkaline foods.

Better sleep foods: Cherries, bananas, whole grain toast and oatmeal all release sleep producing brain chemicals.

One cannot think well, love well, sleep well if one has not dined well.

—Virgina Woolf

Grocery store favorites

COTTAGE CHEESE – Friendship brand, 1% fat, no salt added (stated clearly on the label), is our favorite. Good tasting too, but be careful, it's easy to mistakenly buy a "salted" Friendship container of cottage cheese by mistake.

PEANUT BUTTER – Crazy Eddies™. Love his name and the product. Imagine a peanut butter containing just one item, peanuts! Joseph's™ Crunchy Valencia peanut butter and a Whole Foods™ brand are other good choices.

CRACKERS – Triscuit's™ "Hint of Salt" is a tasty, crunchy cracker. Finally, a giant food company bakes something that's fun to chew and helps you go. Low in fat, low in salt, low incholesterol. High in satisfaction.

TABATCHNICK™ LOW SODIUM frozen soups are tasty and healthful. These soups come in blue containers. They are an excellent source of protein and fiber. Low salt vegetable and lentil soups are better for you than pizza or pasta, and virtually all foods that begin with the letter "p".

Coffee is a powerful food that does some good when used properly. It is a disease fighter, a stimulant, and changes moods. People who drink coffee weigh less than those who don't. It has zero calories, and speeds metabolism even while not exercising. The caffeine in coffee stimulates the brain and provides energy for longer workouts or walks. Coffee may lower the risk of diabetes and Parkinson's disease, and may improve a sour mood.

However, being a stimulant, the caffeine in coffee is an addictive drug that creates mood swings. Caffeine is a powerful stimulant that can prevent us from knowing which foods work well, and which ones don't. When caffeine represses thought patterns and attitudes, it can mask the effects of our eating. We may not know whether our energy comes from the food, or the coffee.

Coffee can make you feel wired, nervous and edgy at times when feeling calm could serve you better. While it may suppress appetites in the short run, food cravings do increase during the course of the day. Excessive use of coffee can be harmful. Adding sugar and cream makes coffee a calorie rich beverage that prevents us from being thin.

If you wonder whether you're addicted to coffee, see what happens when you try to stop drinking it for two or three days. If you want to quit a coffee addiction, cut back slowly. Dieters should avoid caffeine in the morning. A cup of coffee after lunch is ok, but take your coffee with water, as do Europeans. Drinking water with coffee is easier on the stomach.

Only Irish coffee provides in a single glass all four essential food groups: alcohol, caffeine, sugar and fat.
—Woody Allen

There is no trouble so great or so grave that cannot be diminished by a nice cup of tea.
—Bernard Heroux

If you wish to grow thinner, diminish your dinner.
—H.S. Leigh

Behavioral tip: Slow eaters tend to weigh less than rapid ones. Fast eaters are likely to be overeaters. Slow down!

Green tea: Ounce for ounce, few beverages contain as many health benefits as green tea. Green tea has half the caffeine of coffee, and contains fat burning oxidants. Women who drank tea for 14 years weighed less than those who didn't drink tea. Though there is enough caffeine in a cup of regular tea to cause insomnia if taken around bed-time, tea isn't considered an addictive food. Decaf has as many health properties as regular tea. Make time for tea. Weigh less. Be thin.

Why does man kill? He kills for food. And not only food; frequently there must be a beverage.

—Woody Allen

Food additives

Let's face it, food makes us happy. It reduces stress and gives us a temporary sense of satisfaction and comfort. Food is a necessity for life, so why shouldn't it make us happy? But some of us tend to become too happy with overly joyful waistlines. Certain food neurons in our brains can act in a dreadfully misguided way. Food additives can inflate our joy of eating and lead to addictive eating habits.

Why do pizza, chocolate, nachos, and ice cream find their way into our thoughts more often than healthy foods? Why don't we ever seem to crave broiled chicken, steamed broccoli, fresh fish, or fruit? Isn't it strange that we crave foods that are high in calories, fat, sugar and artificial flavors? You may have already guessed the answer – because they taste good.

And you're right. But let's ask ourselves why these foods taste so good. The closer a particular food is to its natural state, the less likely we are to crave it. This is valuable knowledge to have in the fight against food cravings.

Processed foods cause weight problems, making us heavier, depressed and dependent on them. We crave comfort foods as a way to fight the depression that they caused in the first place. Then they drain our willpower to do anything about it. It's a vicious cycle. The key to becoming thin lies in finding our way out of the artificially induced prison of emotionally driven eating.

The bottom line is many foods are drugs, and most of us have become addicted to them. We are food addicts who buy our legal drugs at grocery stores. Our addictions are not very different from addicts who buy heroin, cocaine, alcohol, tobacco, etc. In order to break free, we need to know why certain foods act as drugs in our bodies. We need to detoxify our way to healthful eating.

There are over 3,000 approved food additives in America. Almost all packaged foods contain some of them. They are chemicals that change the natural properties of our food. Most are designed to make food look and taste better. Preservatives are additives that keep bacteria from growing on food. They also increase the shelf life of food products. The following food additives have especially undesirable side effects:

Artificial sweeteners: NutraSweet is found in 5,000 different food products. It's listed in 600 different medicines, including many children's medicines. Other artificial sweeteners include Sweet-n-Low™, Splenda™, Tagatose™, and Neotame™. Whenever you eat something sweet that has zero calories, your body reacts by increasing its cravings for the missing sugar calories.

Fake sweeteners are just a marketing gimmick. They give you the short-term satisfaction of having sweets without the guilt, but the long-term effect will keep you buying more artificial sweeteners. Those who use sugar substitutes end up eating more than if they were eating foods that contained real sugar. It's a win-win situation for the food manufacturers, and we lose. These "products" have been used as food additives for over 20 years. Knowing the effect of artificial sweeteners, it's no surprise that America's weight problems have worsened over the last 20 years. Studies point to an addictive quality in artificial sweeteners. Diet soda is loaded with artificial sweeteners. Now there is a support group for diet soda addicts offering tips on how to detoxify from the addiction.

Sugar

Refined sugar is present in nearly all processed foods, and goes by many names: dextrose, glucose, maltose, corn syrup, etc. Americans consume about 200 pounds of sugar per year – about half a cup per day. Over the years, consumption of sugar additives has increased in proportion to our weight problems. One study discovered 76 ways that sugar can damage long-term health.

In addition to making us fatter, excessive sugar consumption causes increased fatigue, arthritis, migraines, lower immune system functioning, gallstones, gum disease and heart disease. Recently it was discovered that cancers inside the body choose sugars for maintenance and growth. Cancer cells appear to enjoy eating sugar as much as we do. Another study found that sugar is more addictive than cocaine. When given the choice, cocaine addicted lab rats chose sugar over cocaine.

Of all food additives, sugar is our most difficult challenge. It's the major reason dieters fail to permanently lose weight. Not only is sugar available and delicious, it is a substance that's as addictive as any we know of.

There is hope for us, an effective treatment and cure for sugar addiction, and it comes from an old friend, Mother Nature. Eating natural foods is the quickest way to detoxify our bodies from processed sugar. Natural foods restore our bodies to a more balanced metabolism and slowly decrease sugar cravings. By freeing ourselves of sugar addiction, we will have more energy and better mental health.

Salt

This assault on salt could save your life (see the "how to make a miracle" story at end of the book). Salt may be an even bigger health menace than sugar. In 2011, about 100,000 Americans will die of salt related disease. Excessive consumption of salt contributes to high blood pressure, strokes, heart disease, kidney disease and fluid retention. Salt draws water into our bloodstreams increasing the volume of blood. This forces the heart to work harder than it should. Often the result is congestive heart failure.

The American Heart Association (AMA) has been campaigning to reduce the amount of salt in packaged and restaurant foods by 25 percent over five years. Some food companies are going along with this plan, but it's not enough. We need to cut back dramatically on salt, and we need to do it now. Good health demands that we not wait five years, or even five days. Middle age Americans who reduce salt intake by as little as 30% are 1/4 less likely to suffer heart attacks or stroke.

We need about 500 mg of sodium per day. Millions of us consume 3,000 mg or more. The less salt you eat the better your health will be. Excess salt that we eat is hidden in processed foods like tomato sauce, canned soups, condiments and other jarred and canned products. Just about everything sold off a store shelf contains salt – even bread. Only a small fraction comes from the salt you add to food at home. Salt is addictive. Companies load it into foods to keep you coming back for their food products, and possibly for no other reason. A McDonald's double cheeseburger contains about 1,150 mg of sodium all by itself, over twice the amount you need in a day. Frozen dinners often contain over 700 mg. Even a bowl of raisin bran may contain 300 mg of salt.

Is there any real difference between salted candy and filtered cigarettes? Both products will love us to death if we allow it. Unfortunately, both will continue to be sold legally long after we're gone.

The good news is that we know our taste for salt can change quickly. Food containing much less salt will improve in flavor after just a couple of low-salt days. You can reduce your salt consumption and extend your life, by yourself, for yourself and your family. Here's how.

Carefully examine food labels. Don't buy products that add salt, MSG or baking soda. Search out and buy foods containing "no added salt" on the label.

Replace salt with herbs and other spices. Make friends with Mrs. Dash™ and other salt-free products that contain healthful herbs and spices. Use seasoned vinegars instead of salt and buy sodium free chicken broth for added flavor. Before eating canned tuna, rinse and drain much of the sodium away. If you think sea salt is better than regular sodium, think again. Sea salt contains over 80% of the same ingredients as table salt.

Eat potassium rich foods to reduce the effect of salt on your blood pressure. Potassium is abundant in bananas, dried apricots, baked beans, cantaloupe, skim milk, orange juice, baked potato and raisins. Eating three or four times more potassium than salt will help you maintain a healthy blood pressure.

Sodium nitrates are preservatives added to foods such as bacon, corned beef, ham, lunch meats, sausage, pepperoni and hot dogs. They prevent the growth of bacteria and also give meat a pink color that makes it appear healthier than it really is. Nitrates are considered dangerous by the FDA, but haven't been banned due to their ability to prevent spoilage and botulism.

Eating processed meat increases the risk developing cancer. The American Institute for Cancer Research recommends that we completely avoid processed meats. Americans eat 20 billion hot dogs a year; about 70 hot dogs per person. Eating just one ounce of processed meat a day increases our risk of stomach cancer.

MSG™: Most people associate MSG with Chinese food. But MSG is a flavor boosting additive found in nearly all processed food and fast food restaurants. It is used by food manufacturers to enhance flavors and can lead to food addiction. Just because a food label doesn't mention MSG by name, means nothing. it could be listed by another name. Beware of food labels that list "natural flavorings" or "spices" as these are legal terms for MSG.

In the 1960s, scientists learned that MSG produced undesirable health issues and obesity. Alarms have been raised and the food industry was pressured to remove MSG from baby food. However, the FDA has never legally prohibited the use of MSG in American baby food. The FDA has refused to consider any research that suggests that MSG is unsafe for the American food supply.

One of MSG's effects is to trigger a sharp increase in insulin production. This leads to fat storage and a "food craving" response. One way to test this is to make a short list of the foods you crave and then check their labels. With a little research, you will find that many of them contain MSG, but it isn't always easy to identify. MSG is present in the following ingredients: yeast, gelatin, whey protein, pectin, natural beef flavoring, soy protein stock, enzymes, powdered milk, broth, "seasonings", bouillon, citric acid, malt extract, "flavor" and "flavorings."

MSG can be found in salad dressings, ice cream, cheeses, medications, frozen foods; even chewing gum and cigarettes. MSG causes us to crave foods that make us fatter, when we should be eating a balanced diet of natural foods.

Killer foods (over the long term) include hot dogs, hamburgers, steaks, ribs, meat loaf, pork, mutton, sausage, bacon, spam, cheese, processed meats; foods fried in animal fats; foods with added salt and/or sugar such as chips, pretzels, margarine, donuts, ice cream, sorbet, cake, cookies, cereals, syrups, pie and soft drinks; white bread, white rolls, white rice, white pasta; foods with artificial ingredients.

Portion size tip: If there's no measuring cup around, use your fist to determine the right amount of food. Just about every portion should be about the size of your fist.

WHERE'S THE BEEF? He was 70+ and the multi-millionaire owner of a company that shipped delicious sirloins and T-bones across the nation to restaurants and individuals. From personal experience, the sirloins were superb. However when this prince of sirloin surprisingly accepted our dinner invitation, we served him and his wife wild salmon. I shared some negative heart health news with our successful visitor.

"Fish is fine." His response was quick and sincere. "We eat fish, and we like it. But I could never let a day go by without some meat on the table, and I have as much energy as I ever have – especially since they put in the heart stents" (surgically implanted devices that open up obstructed coronary arteries).

Hey, selling steak is what the man did for a living. Selling cigarettes and cigars is the job of the tobacco guys. Protecting ourselves from their products has to be our assignment. Who else?

The sirloin guy was good at selling steaks for over 35 years. But the steaks that made him wealthy even broke HIS heart. Those thick sirloins continue to break the hearts of countless steak "lovers". Our point is that ravaging our heart with dangerous foods has to end. Stop it!

WORLD'S OLDEST MAN: At age 114, Walter Breuning said he lived as long as he has because he left every meal a little bit hungry and limited his meals to two per day during the previous 35 years of his life. "You should push back from the table when you're still hungry."

Breuning eats a big breakfast and lunch every day, but no supper. "I have weighed the same (135 lbs., 5'8") for 35 years, and that's about the way it should be. You get in the habit of not eating at night and you realize how good you feel. If you could just tell people not to eat so darn much."

Breakfast at Breuning's house, around 8 a.m., usually consisted of eggs, toast, or pancakes. "I eat a lot of fruit every day." He also takes a baby aspirin. "Just one baby aspirin, that's the only pill I ever take, no other medicine."

And he drinks lots of water. "I drink water all the time plus coffee. I drink a cup and a half of coffee for breakfast and a cup with lunch." The world's oldest man has been healthy his entire life and believes diet played a large part of it.

"Everybody was poor years ago. When we were kids we ate what was on the table. Crusts of bread or whatever it was. You ate what they put on your plate, and that's all you got." He believes that working hard has helped extend his life. "Work never hurt anybody."

Breuning's last job ended at age 99. On eating out: "Once you get used to not eating in restaurants, you don't want to anymore."

If you want to cheat death and the aging process, consider the following: Eat fish taken from cold ocean waters. Fish will keep your DNA in good shape because of omega-3 fatty acids. Salmon may be best. A low stress lifestyle, plus nutritional foods will keep you younger, especially if you're not a couch potato.

Make and maintain friendships. People with close friends live longer than loners. Cut visits to restaurants to no more than one a month. Preparing meals and eating at home allows for better quality control of foods, and less salt, sugar, fat in you. Live on top of a mountain. Residents atop the Swiss Alps have fewer heart problems than those below, perhaps because they get more sunshine and vitamin D. Breathe cleaner air and live longer.

DENTAL PERFECTION

The first thing I do in the morning is brush my teeth and sharpen my tongue.

—Dorothy Parker

A man loses his illusions first, his teeth second, his follies last.

—Helen Rowland

You don't have to brush your teeth, just the ones you want to keep.

—Unknown

She laughs at everything you say. Why? Because she has fine teeth.

—Benjamin Franklin

Sick teeth and gums are linked to sick hearts and brains. Proper heart care, brain care and dental care are collectively important. Here's how to keep your teeth and gums healthy forever. After one final treatment time, you may manage your mouth forever without being x-rayed, examined, or drilled by dentists.

First, fix your teeth and gums perfectly one final time to establish a healthy dental baseline. Make an appointment at a school of dentistry or dentist. By the time you're dentally ok, you'll know how to keep your teeth and gums healthy by yourself. This chapter is about how pleasant life can be without having mouth or teeth drilled, needled, dug into, capped, x-rayed, pulled.

Some tortures are physical and some are mental, but the one that is both is dental.

—Ogden Nash

Follow these guidelines for dental health perfection:

FLOSS nightly before you sleep. If you have time, floss after breakfast too. Flossing plus using a water jet and toothpicks, provide maximum removal of decay causing bacteria. If the invisible devils in all mouths have their way and get to hang around overnight to enjoy unbothered sex, hey multiply 30 times by morning. Then they breakfast on tooth enamel and gum surfaces. You don't want that.

Use un-waxed floss unless the spacing between your teeth is too tight. In that case, waxed floss is indicated, though it could seal food particles further into gums, not a good thing. Flossing is about scraping plaque off teeth and extracting food particles hiding underneath gums and between teeth. Oral B™ brand ultra dental floss is worth a try. Unlike other floss products, it's made out of spongy nylon fibers that stretch thin to fit easily into tight spaces between teeth. It flicks away plaque. Guide floss between your teeth using a gentle rubbing motion against the sides. Do not snap the floss. When the floss reaches the gum line, gently slide it into the space between the gum and tooth and flick it upward. Hold the floss tightly against the tooth, rubbing it from the gum with upward motions.

Those who floss daily live longer than those who don't. Men with gum disease have a whopping 70 percent higher risk of developing heart disease. Another good thing happens because of flossing: Our breath improves, increasing chances for more kissing, cuddling, and fooling around.

Water jetting

Water jetting is an important dental procedure that too many of us know too little about. If you live with teeth and gums in your mouth, using a water jet after meals is more important than just about anything else, including brushing. It's at least as necessary as flossing. Using a jet daily enables your gums to feel like nature intended, and not bleed.

A water jet works quickly, safely, effectively. It forces food particle harboring bacteria out from between teeth and from below the gum line. It massages and strengthens gums, improving blood circulation. The jets work by delivering water at a pressure of hundreds of pulses per minute. The combination of water pressure and pulsation removes debris and bacteria. Not bad for a device that costs about $50, considerably less than the $100+ for a single professional cleaning, exam, etc. When you combine the benefits of a water jet with flossing and tooth picking, and eat healthfully, dental problems may leave you alone permanently.

Dentists prosper because about 80% of Americans don't floss or use a water jet during teeth cleaning. Some say caring for teeth takes too much time. Others either forget or are too lazy to floss. The result is that dental disease has become a national epidemic, right alongside obesity. Let's join the 20 percent who make the effort to maintain mouths with healthy teeth and gums.

Corporate mischief: Some of the water jet folks boast that their product works better than dental floss. That's deceptive marketing at best. Floss and water jets go between our teeth to remove food particles. But they clean the same oral areas differently. Use both and you will achieve better results. Floss scrapes out small, sticky food particles that a Jet could miss. Jets can expel particles that floss doesn't catch. They complement each other and shouldn't be considered competitive products. Use these products (floss, water jet, toothpicks, toothbrush) to enjoy oral health.

Water jetting benefits:

- Gums get massaged and stimulated. Gum health is restored. Bleeding stops. Jetting takes little time.
- Food particles and bacteria hiding between teeth and below the gum line are removed safely. Gum disease is far less likely.
- Our breath freshens.
- A portable water jet will go to work with you.
- Warm water and/or mouthwash can be used.
- Braces are not disturbed by a water jet.

THE TOOTHPICK, like floss and jets, cleans around the gum area and between teeth. Try Doctors Tooth Picks™. Toothpicks should not replace flossing or water jetting. When you use these three dental tools, and brush your teeth properly, your oral health is pretty much assured so long as you don't eat sticky or sugary foods.

BRUSHING: Brush at least twice a day, after breakfast and before you go to sleep. Keep an extra toothbrush + paste next to your portable water jet at work. Your toothbrush should have SOFT nylon bristles and round ends. Medium and hard bristles wear down tooth enamel. ORAL B™ brand sells only soft bristle toothbrushes. Better yet, buy a power toothbrush with rotation oscillation for about $20 and clean your teeth and gums quicker, probably better.

Night time dental perfection:

- Use a tooth pick to scrape away plaque between teeth at the gum line. – 2–3 minutes
- Floss to remove plaque and food particles lodged between teeth and gums. – 3–4 minutes
- Use your water jet to expel remaining food particles. – 2 minutes
- Brush with toothpaste to polish your teeth. Remember to brush the tongue and the roof of your mouth. – 2 minutes

> *The devil fears the Word of God, but can't bite it.*
> *It breaks his teeth.*
>
> —Martin Luther

MIRACLES & MORE

Down and up in the Big Apple

by Hannah Davis

New York City! What the; wwwhhhyyy? That was the reaction of friends in my small North Carolina hometown when I told them I was moving. I was meant to be in NYC. It's where dreams come true, where I was going to "make it" as an actress. What else? Does anyone move to New York unless they want to act professionally, be a musician, or make big money on Wall Street? I learned that soon after arriving and meeting other "new" people.

To make it as an actress, you need connections, you need the look, and talent (in that order). I believed I had tons of talent, so making connections was the next step. To me, having "the look" means being in really great shape. I needed to work on that one.

I maintained a healthy lifestyle in college in North Carolina, and New York seemed like the perfect setting for staying on track. Walking up and down subway stairs and rushing to cross streets to avoid aggressive motorists burned lots of calories, plus frequent gym workouts. I dropped pounds from the brisk walking alone. Everyone in NY walks fast.

I took a job as a nanny to pay the bills while I looked for acting work. It was either that or bar tending. Working late at night was not conducive for getting eight hours of quality sleep. I needed great skin without under-eye baggage. That comes with good sleeping habits.

My job as a nanny came with perks like free food. "Starving actor" would not describe me. I had whatever foods I wanted. Eating was just a reach away, and I took and took, then took some more. Between Eli's Bread Factory and eating children leftovers in addition to my own meal, the battle to just say "no" and act on it was being lost. I put on pounds. You know it's not good for you when it's free, it's sitting right there, and you take it. I had the perfect set-up for becoming overweight.

In addition to this challenge, I faced the constant hustle and bustle of daily life in the city. I would just grab food on the go instead of cook at home. So much of NYC culture is centered around eating. There is that new restaurant, the happy hours, and fast food dining with friends. It was a challenge to maintain the right weight, but still have some food fun.

Most of all I needed discipline. A chunky actress doesn't get work. I decided to cheat two meals a week to keep from going crazy from being totally obsessed with what I could and couldn't eat. Notice, the word is "meal" not an entire day of cramming junk into my face. That could easily ruin an entire week of healthy eating. It's far easier to eat 3500 calories (equal to a pound) than it is to burn it. However, the muscle you put on from weight lifting does spike your resting metabolic rate so it's not too hard to stay in shape when you do allow for "cheat" meals.

Even when I cheat, I try to make the smartest bad decision possible. For example, if I want to drink, I will choose either a low calorie vodka and club soda with lime, or if I have some calories to spare, a glass of red wine for antioxidant power. For a cheat meal. if a bacon cheeseburger comes with a side of fries, a side salad or steamed veggies substitutes for the fries.

If I have a busy week ahead, I try to take time on Sundays to cook meals to carry with me through the week. I believe this extra effort saved my shape. It is a bumpy ride and I fall off the right food wagon from time to time, but I try to keep a focus on the bigger picture, being thin and healthy.

Not long after arriving in New York, I got booked for a TV appearance on the daytime soap, All My Children. I wanted to look my best to fit in with the "stars." To be as tiny as Susan Lucci, the actress who played Greenlee at the time, I would need to work out more often (which was ok) and try to live on about 1000 calories a day (not going to happen). Balance is a good thing for me. Exercising for the health benefits in addition to eating well make me happier than trying to fit in with daytime soap stars. Soon I told the casting director goodbye.

Becoming an NFL cheerleader was on my "to do" list. Not only do I love football and know a lot about it, I love to dance. When you see Jet cheerleaders in uniform, you know that looking great and feeling great in your own skin are two prerequisites for the job. I exercised with weights, did 20 minutes of cardio 2–3 days a week. I trained to become more flexible, quicker, and learn dance routines. I also spent hours stretching and learning how to do a split, something I'd never before been able to do. To make the Jets cheerleader squad, you have to do splits.

After months of training came the tryouts. I made it past the first round of freestyle dance. I then passed the second round of choreographed dancing and performing in a kick line. The third round had me answering questions like, "can you tell me about a current event?". The finals were held a week later and out of the 40 women who made it to finals, 25 made the team. I didn't, but I had learned how to do those damn splits.

Next I worked for a talent agency, the "other side" of the entertainment business. Office hours from 8 a.m. to 8 p.m., sometimes later. No time to exercise. And instead of walking around the city, I sat behind a desk, producing a shock to my physical and emotional systems. About a year into this job, I was more stressed, more emotional and more frustrated. I had a breakdown. An anxiety attack forced me to re-evaluate my life and decide what I really wanted to do with it.

More than anything I wanted to be happy. That's all. What makes me happy? Beyond helping maintain weight, exercise helps me sleep better. My mood improves. I wanted to be happy and also I wanted to help others avoid an anxiety attack on an office stairwell in New York.

Why not make a career out of exercising and teaching others how to do it? This wonderful solution screamed into my face every time a friend asked me what they should be doing. Every time I was in the gym I felt like creating a new exercise move.

After graduating from The Academy of Personal Training and working at a gym for a year, I established my own training business under the name, Body by Hannah. I trained high profile clients including the editor-in-chief of a woman's health magazine and the CEO of Jones Apparel Group. I contributed to magazines and health blogs and even made it back on TV, this time to show off exercise skills. I am happy.

Among my challenges as a trainer are to correct posture affected by too much time hunching over a computer; reverse the effects of being overweight; and correct muscle imbalances caused by repetitive movements. To see a client successfully lose weight simply by becoming more active and eating right is like witnessing a miracle. The transformation is beautiful. To see energy restored and physical strength increase is like helping construct an improved version of the same person.

I have a great job, but you don't need to be a personal trainer to inspire others into a life of fitness. Transform your life and invite someone to exercise with you while you are doing it. Going "there" with a friend will keep you both on track.

—Hannah Davis is an independent personal trainer in New York City. Visit her at www.BodyByHannah.com.

Fall and recovery

by Charles (Chaz) William Glunk II

I am a professional ballet dancer. It is easy to assume that the life of a dancer is all glamour and glitz. Unfortunately that assumption is far from the truth. The life of a dancer is wrought with uncertainty, stress and doubt. Everything beneath the spotlight casts a shadow and the light of the stage can burn so bright that it is blinding. In the resulting blindness, the darkness can be all consuming. So I ask, on your darkest day, how do you find the courage to look into the light? For several years, I contemplated this question. How can people treat someone with such little concern?

It was time to face the truth and most importantly, face myself. I came to a realization that the gradual unraveling of my self-image, my confidence, my self-awareness was due to bullying. The resulting depression had brought upon my downfall. Six years into my professional ballet career, I struggled. I made a very modest amount of money for 26 to 32 weeks a year and it was starting to take its toll both physically and mentally. In time, the constant financial burden of student loans, health insurance, credit card debt, and day to day living expenses began to affect my love of dance.

The answer seemed to fall from the sky when my best friend at the time, who left the ballet company in South Carolina for a show in Las Vegas, suggested that I follow her out west. This idea tempted me with the notions of steady pay, comfortable work conditions, health insurance, and of course the glitter and glam that the pre-housing crisis Las Vegas offered. I felt set free, like a caged bird taking flight for the first time after captivity. Before I knew it, I was packing my little Ford Focus hatchback to the point of exploding at the seams. I was behind the wheel of "Little Lizzie" and singing at the top of my lungs, heading west on I-40.

The Las Vegas Strip is a city known to be built on a foundation of money, tourism, sex, booze, and greed. The strip is also built on the notions of prosperity and good luck. Tourists come from all over the world to pit their odds against the house. Some come empty handed and leave with opulence. Others come heavy-laden with opulence and walk away empty-handed. In some ways, that's the thrill of going to Las Vegas. It was certainly a similar thrill with which I fueled my personal dream of success. Within two days of arrival, the hotel at which my friend was employed as a dancer had an open audition. At the heart of the strip, I auditioned and danced all over the house odds. It's as if every ornate, flashing bulb was a spotlight shining solely for me and within the confines of the decadent walls and flashing signs, Finally, I could have financial stability and not have to give up dance.

Something went wrong. It was on a level that I'd either ignored or simply been blind to for the first six months. It started with teasing me for signs of aging. Age is a dancer's worst enemy, but it quickly became more personal. It became commonplace to tease me, even on stage, all fun and games until someone gets hurt. I tried to rise above the comments. I bottled up the pain deep inside me. Yet somehow, by not engaging in their juvenile games of cat and mouse, the comments grew harsher and crueler. A certain group in particular began setting out daily to make me an outcast. They wanted me to feel like I didn't belong. Every moment, even beneath the spotlight, was under the shade of their teasing. They were carnivores eating away at my self confidence and psyche. The attacks grew to the point that when I look back upon these dark days, I grow increasingly embarrassed that I let these people say such cruel things. I didn't want trouble and, besides, I wasn't one of the "favorites" of the company. If anything, I thought my quiet suffering would help in the end.

In classical dance training, part of stage etiquette is that a performer never speaks on stage unless they are asked. My fellow co-workers had loosely adhered to this. Gestures and noises had been directed at me, however nothing as blatant as what was to come. The attacks grew exponentially. It was no longer only off-stage comments and on-stage gestures. Now, I had to listen to belittling comments in front of 2,000 people. It was hell. I continued to deal with it by bottling up my emotions and drowning my pain with substance. I lived in a fantasy-land. But the bottle inside was beginning to crack. So was my psyche. I didn't think things could get worse. I was wrong.

Long before Vegas became a twinkle in my eye, my mother had been ill. An advanced lung disease was the culprit. My mother was dependent on oxygen to breathe at 47. I'd run from this for years. Suddenly, in the depth of winter, with Christmas only weeks away, my mother's ailing health took a turn for the worse.

Sometimes , when we're clawing our way up through the darkness toward the light, we miss the small points of light available to guide our path. We're blinded by the fury of our actions. This is what almost happened to me. After being surrounded by so much negative energy for so long, I forgot what it felt like to experience something positive. With the power of my family coming together to support my mother, I saw a glimmer of light.

During this crisis, one night stands out. The doctor pulled the family into a private room to talk. He was trying to prepare us for the worst. I was lost. I felt helpless. I felt angry. That night I held my mom's hand and remembered the good times and even some of the bad ones. I cherished every moment and mourned their passing. However, the winds of lament unfurled the sails of change and something deep within me broke free. A new state of mind burst through the fog of my sorrow.

It didn't seem significant then. How could it, really? I'm no fortune teller. All that I remember is visualizing *for* her, holding her tiny hand within mine and concentrating on how strong she was. I sent as much positive energy as I could. Where this energy came from was a mystery to me, but it didn't really matter. I visualized giving her my lungs. I visualized giving her my life. I won't claim responsibility. I can't. However I can say that the next morning both my mother and I began to recover. She began to recover her health. I began to recover my hope. What had been a mustard seed of hope had sprung into a massive and powerful force and things were falling into place for a much brighter future.

It was a hot July. I had a birthday on the horizon. A themed birthday party was to be thrown in my honor. Yes, I was to be the lucky recipient of a "white trash" birthday party. My fellow cast members were happy to jeer and poke fun at the socio-economic class of my origin. I learned the depth of my situation. Now entire groups of people were organizing events to make me feel horrible.

I felt utterly alone, trapped in my own embarrassment, self-disgust, and pity. Fortunately, I was never really alone. I had a wonderful lover and his excellent family for support. They were holding me tight, not letting me fall. Still, very close to giving up on everything, I decided to place passive behavior in the back seat. I seized life by the horns, and made it mine again. I answer big questions of the "why", "who", and "what" of life with yoga, the perfect union of energy and movement.

Through yoga, I began to learn about energy and the flow of Chi. Through the learning of life's energies, I began to mold my life with this new understanding. I am capable of surrounding myself with the once nameless, positive energy that I discovered. I step forward looking toward the light. I project myself toward the positive things in life, loving what I do have, being thankful for who I am, and looking forward to where I'm going.

I continued to restructure my life from the inside out, leaving Vegas for Sarasota and a job with my first dance teacher. I am enjoying my love of ballet and I love teaching. While working in the studio, I am apprenticing in the ancient art of Yoga. Here I can help others find the good in life to help guard them from the negative. I help people explore their potential through movement, channeling energy, and physical fitness. I have fallen only to recover brighter, happier, and more positive than ever before.

The gift of balance

by Amanda Main

Ten years ago, as I laid in my first savasana (a relaxing posture intended to rejuvenate body, mind, spirit), I knew I had found something that would change my life. At that time, I was a 30-year-old woman, four years sober from alcohol and drugs. In the three years prior, I met the man who was to become my husband and we had two children together. I immediately became a stay-at-home mom who smoked cigarettes, drank coffee and took antidepressants.

I met a woman at a local park who had a child the same age as my oldest. As we watched the kids play, she told me about a local gym with babysitting. She said they had a great yoga class and that she went three times a week. I was very excited about the notion of having a break from my children for an hour and a half three times a week. I truly loved them (and still do) with all my heart, but I was losing it and tired of asking family for favors and then having to listen to what they had to say about my life.

I decided to quit smoking and use the money to pay for the gym membership. With the financials figured out, I started a yoga practice that opened up a new world to explore. As my body became stronger, so did my mind. I loved being in meditation and began to integrate that aspect into my daily life. My circumstances did not change but my outlook did. I became much more comfortable with my life. My relationships deepened as a result and I began to feel joy.

At 28, I became pregnant and all hell broke loose. I couldn't stop eating! I ate from the minute I woke up until the minute I went to bed. I was a cliche. I would send my husband to the local diner for chocolate bread pudding at midnight.

At visits to the gynecologist, he would laugh and say, "You must be having a really good time", never warning me to take this more seriously. By the time I gave birth, I had gained close to 75 pounds.

I was in shock that the baby only weighed seven pounds. I was also in shock that a month later, I hadn't lost the weight. I was faced with a dilemma. Not only was I a new mother with no idea of how to take care of a baby, I was also a new wife. As a new wife, I wanted to look good for my husband, but I had eaten my way to obesity and no longer had the excuse of being pregnant.

Luckily for me but sad for my body, when my daughter was five months old, I became pregnant again. This time I did better. I still gained to the upper end of the scale but not nearly as much. The truth is that I have never returned to my pre-baby weight and don't know if I ever will.

My children are 10 and 11 now. I feel like something changed physiologically in my body when I put on that ridiculous amount of weight. The practice of yoga has helped me to not only accept my body and all of the wonderful things it does, but to really love my body and appreciate the magic that happens when I exercise and eat good food.

As I began to introduce foods to my children, I started to pay attention to what exactly I was giving them. I was amazed to learn what was going into commercial foods. I realized that I had to become more comfortable in the kitchen if I was to feed my family healthfully. I spent hours on the internet finding ways to make simple dishes using fresh and local foods. I learned what was best to eat organic and what was ok to eat conventionally grown.

I found sources for meats that didn't contain hormones or antibiotics. I love to sneak spinach into a turkey meat loaf or grind flax seeds and mix them into the bread crumbs for chicken fingers. I am not above being sneaky when it comes to the health of my family. If my children choose not to have a full serving of broccoli, it's ok because there is cauliflower in the mashed potatoes that they don't know about. There are websites that can help you to make the transition from the normal American diet to something better.

You don't have to do a dramatic make over all at once. Start small. Once you begin to integrate these kinds of things, you will want to do more. Websites also offer printable downloads to keep in your wallet of what fish are ok to eat or what produce to buy organic. The most up to date seafood guide is at http://www.montereybayaquarium.org and the produce is available at http://www.foodnews.org. By changing our awareness and attitudes when it comes to food, we begin to eat better and excess weight will fall off.

Something else paramount not only in eating properly, but to my life in general is meditation practice. I discovered meditation through yoga. It is the single most important thing I do on a daily basis. I started with just five minutes a day. Anyone can do something for five minutes.

Start by focusing on your breaths (count them on the inhale or the exhale, or observe them (depth, speed, impact on your stomach, lungs, head, etc.) and see where it takes you. Meditation has allowed me to see my strengths. It has given me a canvas on which I create the life of my dreams.

Although I still drink coffee, I believe meditation has helped me to get and stay off antidepressants and cigarettes. It has allowed me to live a life as a sober woman with balance and grace and for that I will be happy to help others discover its magic.

I truly believe we can eat ourselves into good health or we can eat ourselves to death. The choice is ours.

—Amanda Main teaches meditation at ReFlex Arts in Sarasota, FL where she's also a massage therapist. Contact her at www.balanceforliving.com.

How to make your very own miracle

by Shane

PARANORMAL is defined as something that happens outside the range of normal experience or scientific explanation. The scientific community generally does not support what is characterized as the paranormal. But over half of Americans believe in psychic/spiritual healing.

I'm not a cheerleader for science anymore, especially when it hurts, and doesn't heal us. Being receptive to any paranormal happenings in our lives is more fun, and occasionally a lot less scary.

The angel of death is a concept that has existed since the beginning of history. In English speaking nations, this Angel is known as the grim reaper. One of his assignments is to escort the deceased to the afterlife. Grandpa called this Angel "Uncle Jerry" and feared him mightily, as do I. Jerry also purportedly causes death from time to time, so bribing or tricking or outwitting him in order to extend life seems like a good idea.

At age 65 in 2005, I was living in the valley of the Shadow of Death. Cancers and heart disease depressed many of the retired folks who lived along Sanibel Way in Bradenton, FL, me included. Our fears competed with noisy parties as to what would dominate the neighborhood on any given day. The bus that Uncle Jerry drives picked up two neighbors in July. I knew Jerry was driving up my driveway when I felt the fading breath/sounds of a dying man, me.

Coughing was continual. I couldn't sleep. My heart raced to an irregular and rapid rhythm. Breaths were shallow and got weaker amidst fits of coughing. My chest was sore, achy, and hurt a lot. Nonstop coughing alone taught me what it's like to dance with death; intimate as hell but no fun. Moving beyond the toilet ten feet away became too long of a trip.

"Shane see a doctor," demanded a son, a girlfriend and a wise Latino nurse from across the street who prepared chicken soup and delivered it lovingly. After a month of misery I went to the doctor who quickly declared me to be a medical mess; congestive heart failure, atrial fibrillation, enlarged heart and blood pressure so high it was out-of-sight. I was, he said, close to being worse off than dead.

Worse than dead.... hmmm, how could THAT be? When you stroke out, the doctor explained, it can be. "Listen Shane, go to the hospital. You've got serious problems that I can't treat. I'll send over specialists to take care of you."

I didn't go to the hospital. A few weeks later a mini stroke arrived as predicted. It caught my attention enough to consult with a cardiac/stroke specialist in Sarasota. He wanted to operate the next day, a "minor" procedure that would normalize my heartbeat. After that, he wanted me to take eight heart/stroke pills a day for the rest of my life. These included Warfarin™, a blood thinner also used to kill rats.

When my favorite nurse told me about the rat killer, I snatched back control of my medical destiny from the stroke expert. I turned down the surgery and six of the eight pills he wanted to prescribe. "Shane take the Warfarin. It's what you need."

Not the right advice. If my health and life got screwed up even worse, let it be all my fault. It's my body, live, die, or linger in a situation worse than death. Anyway, to me death wasn't worse than taking rat poison to thin my blood. Something better had to be out there, or just let me die.

Have the courage to live. Anyone can die.
—Robert Cody

Death is one appointment we must keep, but for which no time is set.
—Charlie Chan

If this is dying, I don't think much of it.
—Lytton Strachey

For three days after death, hair and fingernails continue to grow,
but phone calls taper off.
—Johnny Carson

The second stroke came two months later. My left arm wouldn't move, scratch, lift, grasp, push the TV remote. The feeling was gone. The arm was indifferent to the rest of me. It just hung there, dead.

Stroke number 3 arrived April 2006 and this event wasn't a cause of celebration either. My ability to speak was replaced with the babbling sounds of an eight-month old. Nor could I read, write, or walk normally. My once brisk gait was replaced by a slow sluggish limp.

Uncle Jerry was closing in again. The short list for bus pick up surely included me. For no particular reason that I remember, I wanted to live longer. I wanted a "just not now" delay on death, so I decided to cash my social security check and flee Florida like a scared kid. Perhaps I could retire in reverse, to the north. But in any case, I wanted to hide somewhere, anywhere away from Uncle Jerry, and that rat poison specialist.

Death is a very dull, dreary affair and my
advice to you is to have nothing to do with it.
—Somerset Maugham

For me, the sunshine state had become God's waiting room. Three loving relatives flew in to pack, load, and deliver me to an apartment on a hilltop near Charlottesville, home of the University of Virginia. This was the summer of 2006 and despite the medical odds, good things began happening. Living outside the valley of the Shadow of Death quickly made a medical difference. I had far fewer concerns in this new neighborhood where all were healthier and younger than me. Even if Uncle Jerry found me on that hill in Virginia, a pretty student nurse would hold my hand as I boarded his bus, a reasonably happy ending.

On its own, my left arm returned from its nap, for unknown reasons. Speech returned though the words for several months were as sluggish as my walk. The achy chest and the limp remained, but in Virginia, at least for now, uncle Jerry left me alone.

Except for one semi-famous heart specialist at the University of Virginia, doctors didn't push operations. I took three medicines daily from 2007 until mid 2010; aspirin (made from a tree), Digoxin™ from a backyard plant, and a water pill. There were no discernable side effects.

If you realize that all things change, there is nothing you will try to hold onto. If you are not afraid of dying, there is nothing you cannot achieve.

—Unknown

There are two ways to live your life. One is as though nothing ever is a miracle. The other is as though everything is a miracle.

—Albert Einstein

Miracles happen to those who believe in them.

—Bernard Berenson

What is sacred? Of what is the Spirit made? What is worth living for and what is worth dying for? The answer to each is the same, only love.

—Don Juan deMarco

Miracle: An unexpected event, often thought of as a perceptible interruption in the laws of nature. A wonderful, unlikely but beneficial happening believed caused by a higher power, or a miracle worker.

The first week in Virginia I limped about the downtown area looking for the state wine store. I noticed a tiny medical shop on Main Street. The place looked like it came right out of an episode of the Twilight Zone. Perhaps 50 illnesses were listed (or rather plastered) on the storefront window that could be treated inside. They included heart disease and stroke. I opened the door and walked inside, a decision that led to the restoration of my health.

"Come in. I can help you." Dr. Q. (PhD) was standing in his office alone. He reminded me of Pat Morita, the Mr. Miyagi (mentor/wise man) in the Karate Kid movie. Q's face wore a kind expression. His body posture was confident. I asked him to sell me medicine for my heart and head.

"It doesn't work that way. First you need to be my patient. I find out what's wrong, then you can buy medicine." Being Dr. Q's patient cost $100 for the first exam/treatment, a two hour comprehensive physical/mental work-up, and $50 for each one hour session afterwards. Q was retired, and opened his office to lock boredom out of his life. He intended to treat one or two patients a day just to get out of the house and because "work is good". He was born in Korea.

Unlike the dozens of doctors I met over a lifetime who carried a medical kit containing three of four tools (prescriptions, advice, surgery), Dr. Q's medical toolbox must have totaled over 30.

Special menus were created by Dr. Q to feed my sick heart because "the right food is your best medicine." Acupuncture needles darted into my ear lobes and other parts without bloodshed. Dr. Q literally smashed into smithereens "knots" in my upper back that didn't belong there. Herbs were formulated into medicines and capsulated by him in the office during the appointment. He taught me stand-still workout routines that enable simultaneous TV viewing and exercise.

Background music/chanting promoted healing. Some treatment techniques were so incredible I tended not to believe even as the paranormal stuff was being applied, so I won't pursue that EXCEPT for the miracle(s) Dr. Q predicted and showed me how to make happen. All in all, this retired doctor, born in N. Korea, made conventional American medical practice seem comparatively pathetic.

Some of Q's paranormal techniques were hard to believe, including his instructions on how to make the miracle that restored my health. After four sessions, Dr. Q summarized my medical situation. "Mr. Shane, you're very sick, and I can't help you." (Not a big surprise).

"What now?"

"Find someone to take care of you and love you. SHE will save your life."

Where there is great love, there are always miracles.
—Willa Cather

"No sir, that won't happen. A woman's never taken care of me before, or loved me all that much." (perhaps I took too much time) Dumb response, sick me was arguing with a wise, wonderful man. "Dr. Q, I just moved here. I don't know any woman who would love me." My search for love had come up empty for 44 years (and two failed marriages of 14 years each). Why bother looking for love again at age 66?

Dr. Q persevered. "Ask your relatives. They'll help you find someone."

"They don't live here Dr. Q. Anyway, the ones who would do it are dead."

"Who's your favorite relative?"

"Grandma Gussie. She died about 25 years ago."

"No. She's with you. She wants to help. Go home and ask your grandma to help you."

That night I spoke to Gussie. (How could it hurt?)

"Grandma, it's me, Michael. First of all, I love you. I miss you."

Tears filled my eyes for the first time in years. "I apologize for not contacting you before now. Never crossed my mind I could. No one told me, and I wasn't smart enough to figure it out myself.

"Grandma, I need a favor. My doctor said you will help find a woman to love, someone who will save my life; perhaps someone wonderful like you."

Finally I was more than stupid. "I know you are happy in heaven grandma. Give my love to Betty (my mother), and (sisters) Susan and Rozie."

Dear reader, it's no surprise to you that the next day I found a special someone, smart too (PhD), who saved my life. Finding a wonderful woman so soon after Dr. Q. told me how to do it was a happy development and incredible, but it wasn't a miracle. It was more like winning a lottery, and that happens. We sipped coffee downtown and a week later, we were living together.

This is a health book, so will spare you details of the relationship, but what carried extraordinary good luck into the paranormal and world of miracles is this: The love of my life looked exactly like grandma Gussie when both were age 47. In my view, that simply can't be brushed aside as coincidental.

My health was ok during the first year of our relationship. Then my significant other saved my life, as Dr. Q said she would. Here's what happened.

Before striking, the three previous strokes provided the same specific warning signals; pain in limbs and upper back. When the same pains came again in 2007, I knew stroke #4 was on its way. I told my love to move back home to avoid being part of a serious stroke scene. She was silent for half an hour, then said what would stop the pending stroke from happening, probably liberating me from these brain killers forever.

"I don't want to leave, but before you kick me out, try one more thing. Your food choices contain too much salt. Just cut back on salty foods and let's see what happens." I did. Two days later I was pain free and have remained stroke free since. No one before my darling shared how the mindless consumption of salty foods leads to strokes.

Summarizing: Miracle one was Grandma Gussie finding me the right woman (herself?) less than 24 hours after I asked her to help. Dr. Q's incredible prediction that an as yet unknown "love" would save my life came true; miracle #2. What a doctor!

How can this benefit you? Well, perhaps your favorite grandma can help you. Or ask for a miracle from ANY relative who loves you. Again, how can it hurt? It worked for cynical, skeptical, non-believing me. Since then I lived longer than anyone, including me, thought possible. Could a miracle be out there for you? Why not!

It's May 17, 2011 and I am living in Florida again without the love of my life or even a dog. Trying to stay healthy while living alone has become the latest crap shoot of my life. But taking this risk at 70 is easier than ever. I keep a low profile and wear a hat in case uncle Jerry is out there looking for me, or filling cans of tomatoes with salt for all I know.

But I don't care. I am comforted by the power of Chi; by Dr. Q; by having tasted love late in life; and by Gussie's miracle presence after so many years. I like my odds of hanging out in health and sunshine on this lovely planet for at least a few more years.

My advice to you?

If you need a miracle, ask your grandma!

And in the end, the love you take is equal to the love you make.

—Sir Paul McCartney

No longer taking pills for head or heart, Shane is writing a biography of uncle Jerry.

GIFT...

"Thin You, Thin Me and the Power of Chi" books

...TO THOSE YOU CARE ABOUT.

Call 1-800-BOOKLOG.

Bookmasters will ship books wherever you wish.

MEAL PLANS

BREAKFAST (*Remember to start your day with plenty of water.*)

Option #1: Half a banana and one additional fruit of your choice (apple, pear, orange, etc.) Coffee or herbal tea.

Option #2: Egg white veggie omelet and a slice of whole grain toast, no butter or cheese. Coffee or herbal tea.

Option #3: Peanut butter on rye toast with honey, and an apple. Coffee or tea.

Option #4: Oatmeal with yogurt, fruit and a little honey or maple syrup. Coffee or tea.

Option #5: Sliced banana, cottage cheese and toasted corn tortilla. Coffee or tea.

Option #6: Fruit smoothie: frozen blueberries, vanilla yogurt, banana, skim milk.

LUNCH ideas also work well for breakfast.

Option #1: Tuna or salmon sandwich on whole grain toast, and a side of applesauce, tea or water.

Option #2: Tossed salad with fat free dressing, half a sweet potato, small handful of unsalted nuts and a piece of fruit. Herbal tea or water.

Option #3: 4–6 oz. baked chicken (no skin), hummus and cucumbers on salt free crackers, tea or water.

Option #4: Grilled Alaskan salmon with spinach and yams. Apple slices. Herbal tea or water.

DINNER

Soup's on! Soups are delicious, inexpensive, low calorie, satisfying and easy to prepare. Vegetable and lentil soups are great on a cool day. For more heft in your soup, add a cut-up sweet potato.

DESSERT

Option #1: Small handful of thawed frozen cherries with a scoop of low fat yogurt and half a large banana.

Option #2: Whole grain cereal and fruit.

VITAMINS A daily vitamin/mineral supplement containing calcium and vitamin D can reduce cravings, and may help reduce weight.

> *My doctor told me to stop having intimate dinners for four unless there are three other people.*
>
> —Orson Welles

Coffee calories

	Ounces	Calories
Instant coffee	8	4
Brewed w. 2 tbsp. cream	9	106
Brewed w. 2% milk	9	17
McDonald's Cappuccino	16	130
McDonald's Latte	16	180
McDonald's flavored iced	17	270
Dunkin Donuts Coolatta with cream	16	400
Starbucks Caffe Latte	16	220
Starbucks Peppermint White Chocolate Mocha (whip)	16	560
Baskin Robbins Cappuccino blast	24	480
Dairy Queen Caramel MooLattte	16	630

Junk + fast food

	Calories	Sodium
Burrito with cheese	188	584
Chicken breast sandwich	288	758
Hamburger	300	500
Taco salad	288	886
Roast beef sandwich	346	792
3 pancakes (w.butter & syrup)	519	1103
Hot dog	246	671
Sub sandwich w. cold cuts	456	1650
Baked potato w. cheese	481	701
Fish sandwich w. tartar sauce	431	615
Cheeseburger (double patty)	706	1159
Egg & bacon biscuit	457	999
Vanilla shake (10 oz.)	474	

Fruit calories

Fruit	Calories
Apple (small)	52
Banana (medium)	94
Blueberries (cup)	81
Dates (cup of pitted)	490
Grapefruit (medium)	82
Grapes (cup)	114
Lemon (medium)	17
Cantaloupe, 2.4 oz.	24
Orange (large)	86
Peach (medium)	42
Pear (medium)	98
Strawberries (cup)	46
Watermelon, 10 oz.	92

Vegetable calories

	Serving	Calories
Asparagus	2 oz.	11
Brocolli	3 oz.	35
Kidney beans	3 oz.	108
Cabbage	5 oz.	41
Carrot	1 cup chopped	52
Cauliflower	3.5 oz.	23
Celery	3.5 oz.	14
Corn (kernels)	3.5 oz.	354
Lentils	3.5 oz.	115
Mushrooms	2.5 oz.	20
Onion	3 oz.	36
Peas	3 oz.	72
Potato w. skin	7 oz.	255
Sweet potato, baked	7 oz.	180
Spinach	6 oz.	40
Tomato, raw	2.2 oz.	11